THE MONOLOGUE OF FEAR

FROM DEFEATED AND BROKEN TO POSITIVE AND HOPEFUL

CARLA M. RALSTON

authors
AND CO.

ISBN13: 978-1-913728-19-9

CONTENTS

Foreword vii
Introduction xi

1. The Origins of Fear 1
2. The Supposition of Loss 16
3. The Deterrence of Love 60
4. The Torture of Abandonment 83
5. The Apprehension of Living 105
6. The Uncertainty of Success 126
7. Intimidation of Insanity 142
8. Gathering the Confidence to Ask for Help 160
9. Post-Rehabilitation Adjustment 175
10. PTSD & Epigenetics 193
11. Living Fearlessly 208

About the Author 226

DEDICATION

I would like to dedicate this book to those that have positively changed my life.

I would like to personally acknowledge my dad who I miss dearly, my mom, Tom, Dennis, and Nicole for being there for me when times were difficult.

Thank you for not giving up on me in my weakest moments.

It means more than you will ever know.

FOREWORD

BREAKING DOWN INTERNAL BARRIERS

> *"You are moving so quickly that there is a great deal of fear on the planet, but remember that quite often the fear can be harnessed and used for a singular purpose. You will find yourself in these situations where things seem to be out of control, but do not believe that for a second. You are in much more control than you realize."*
>
> — *STEVE ROTHER & THE GROUP.*

~

WHAT IS FEAR?

Fears exist within all of us. They are constructed by exposure to a frightening situation, person, or object. If there is a belief that something will be dangerous, this may result in a powerful association linked to a negative outcome. When the outcome is consistently affiliated with apprehension or pain, the initial fear becomes solidified. This is a term known as conditioned fear responses. If a stimulus evokes the same response in other similar contexts, it becomes generalized (S. Lissek et al. 2005). From my personal experience, all it takes is one traumatic experience to lead to a long-lasting fear. When events generate these negative associations, memories may provoke post-traumatic stress reactions that impede our ability to adapt to seemingly normal circumstances. However, not all individuals are affected adversely by fear. If the fears do become manifested, avoidance grows, culminating into triggers that threaten the balance of our psyche.

My personal interaction with fear, trauma, and post-traumatic stress disorder has led me to search for resolutions. The hardest part of this journey was unravelling the story behind difficult segments of my life. In order to make a change within myself, I had to be honest about the struggles I have faced. There were so many obstacles as a result of the mental battles I endured. It has taken years to accept myself without passing judgment and imposing doubt.

I had to employ introspection to disengage from maladaptive patterns of thinking. Lessons of greater pertinence came from acknowledging my pain. These fears then became my inner monologue that dictated my thought processes

In order to demonstrate this, I will provide an unfiltered recollection of my life; a no holds barred look into my most devastating and proudest memories. My ultimate dream is to help you manifest great strength from tremendous torment. The stories I will be presenting will not be in accordance with the exact timeline of my life, but rather in an order that corresponds to the theme of each chapter.

References

Lissek, S., Powers, A. S., Mcclure, E. B., Phelps, E. A., Woldehawariat, G., Grillon,

C., & Pine, D. S. (2005). Classical fear conditioning in the anxiety disorders: A meta-analysis. *Behaviour Research and Therapy, 43*(11), 1391-1424. doi:10.1016/j.brat.2004.10.007

Lwempowerment. (2018, January 05). Beacons of Light, February 2017: Awakening the Feminine. https://www.espavo.org/beacons-of-light-february-2017-awakening-the-feminine/

INTRODUCTION

Have you been paralyzed by parts of your past? If so, you are not alone. There are so many of you unable to function normally because one event altered your perspective so much that there's a permanent scar that burns whenever you look at it. Just facing its existence brings your stomach into knots and adrenaline coursing through your veins. Sure, there may be others that feel the way you do, but you still feel entirely alone. You're right, they usually have no clue what you're going through. Because for you, that one moment has dictated who you are in this very moment. You can't live in the present because all you see is what happened, like your worst nightmare, taunting you over and over.

I'm here to tell you that you don't have to live like this. There's a way to process, acknowledge, and escape. This psychological torture has created a brick wall of fear that is difficult to break through. But there is a way to overcome this. I share my story with you in hopes that you can relate to me, re-evaluate your own past, and come with me on this journey to reach your own form of nirvana, peace, and freedom.

I can't promise that you will be one hundred percent better, but I will show you how to put forth an honest effort by learning the tools for success. It is up to you how you implement them. I am your biggest supporter throughout this process. That two-ton elephant that's been sitting on your chest is going to release you from your internal burdens.

I know it seems like an impossible feat. I'm here to guarantee you that it's not. In order to recover from the past, reflection becomes a tool for learning and growth. My strategy is to direct you through the worst experiences of my life, and provide my advice as to how I began to heal. I am not a trained therapist. However, unlike many professionals, I have *lived* and succeeded through the pain. Using my Bachelor's degree in Psychology and specialization in Neuroscience, I will provide a supplementary explanation for my suffering.

The beginning of my book is dedicated to describing the origin of my fears. Subsequently, I will share my early strategies for combating hesitation that impacts interpersonal relationships. I intend to help you rebuild these connections using advice that I considered but never used.

I guess that was because I wanted to believe that people always have the best intentions in friendships. But that is not the case.

After my first fears began to develop, they were reinforced by extensive loss and grief. Because of this, I have been motivated to search deep and wide to find the best solutions to preventing chronic bereavement from destroying the rest of my life. My inspiration has led me to new research on the underlying causes of protracted grief. Using my intimate understanding of loss in combination with what I have learned, I tell you what has worked best for me. In doing so, I hope that you can use my advice to jumpstart your own recovery.

Since the #metoo movement has led to the liberation of many women who endured sexual assault, I have decided to share my story so that silence no longer plagues me. I am speaking out because I know that I am not alone. I believe there are elements of my story that will encourage other females to be brave and fight for justice. There are so many of you that are hurting alone, and I want that to end today. It was not easy for me, but I learned how to rebuild my life. I pray that following my footsteps leads you to a better version of yourself.

In addition to sexual assault, I faced inner conflict, surrounding my feelings of abandonment. The following section is dedicated to expressing how being the daughter of an alcoholic changed me. I will explain how I became a compassionate and supportive family member throughout my dad's addiction. As a result of his troubles, I did not enjoy life. I encourage you to remain positive, however. There is a way to counteract devastation and doubt. Part of that comes with learning that addiction is a disease, not a choice.

Given the tribulations I endured, I genuinely believed I would remain unsuccessful. I was burdened by self-doubt, and therefore, I feared success. In order to generate a newfound sense of self-worth, you must change the way you think. That is a skill I work on emulating throughout this whole process.

Before leaving the distant past, I address recent events that detail my brush with insanity. These two incidents brought me into a mental breakdown and a cycle of vicious addiction. I was so close to not being here to tell my story. I wanted to end my life because my deteriorated mental state and drug use took complete control. But I am standing here today proud of the work I have done to change. My life is dedicated to helping others not only survive their difficult encounters, but also thrive.

Not many succeed without relapse, but I believe that you can. I encourage you to use my personal secrets as a starting point. I created my own strategies for recovery that truly made an impact on me. I am so grateful to share my methods because I believe they will also inspire you to generate success.

Most importantly, these endless cycles of negativity and trauma can be put to an end. Current research in the field of Psychology has provided evidence to support a genetic component to PTSD. Because of this, I believe we can prevent future generations from enduring the same issues. This has led me to propose a framework for developing beneficial coping skills, using my 7-day plan to positivity. Once you take this journey with me, you will no longer be the same person again. You will have the ability to be introspective and truly change. So, let's begin.

1

THE ORIGINS OF FEAR

> *"Nothing in life is to be feared. It is to be understood."*
>
> — *MARIE CURIE.*

So, what am I afraid of? Maybe it's stupid or even crazy, but if I had no fear at all, then I wouldn't be motivated or driven by anything. Everything I intentionally avoid is exactly what I should be running towards. I have to face myself and every construct I've created. Each and every weakness that disables me is also what defines who I am. I didn't always see my life from this perspective, however. I've spent many years avoiding the door that leads to the darkest corners of my mind. Now I realize that I've been lost for a purpose. And that is to acquire the ability to surpass internal crises.

In those moments of despondence, I discovered my inherent purpose. To share this journey with others in hopes that perhaps they too will find their way through pain and suffering. You can become unrestrained from the prison cell inside your mind.

I have a pessimistic mind, however. Everything that should be comforting evokes a sense of negativity and panic. I can clearly visualize what I want to achieve and instead, I stand in the way of my own success. My doubts tell me I am not good enough. I take full responsibility for deferring my dreams, based on the belief they would never escape the confines of my mind. My negative thinking patterns encouraged the transitory relationship between surreal and palpable.

When I was a little girl, I wanted to be a singer, actress, and dancer. I fantasized about becoming a triple threat. I went to dance classes and signed up for music lessons to gain more experience. After building a basic ability to demonstrate my talents, I enrolled in public theatre performances. When it came time to audition, I would perform only what I was comfortable with. Even though I knew I was capable of proving that I could exceed the standards I set for myself, I chose in the pocket melodies bypassing every opportunity to present and sustain notes of power.

I was the confident girl when no one was watching. In

make-or-break moments, I chose to take the easy way out. Those decisions are what set the foundation for my future flights from success. At the time, I genuinely convinced myself that I did my best. Yet in my heart, I knew I cheated myself from truly becoming what I set out to be.

Even later on, I stuck with this dream despite screwing it up for myself on many occasions. It's not as if my parents taught me to be afraid of anything. My mother always encouraged me to believe that I was capable of anything. Every dream that I sought out to chase, she made it possible, working two jobs to support the costs. But more invaluable was the time she spent every day, emotionally building my confidence and always being by my side to help me when I did fail. What was more precious to me was the time she dedicated to me, even when I was capable of accomplishment without guidance. I will always cherish those moments.

My dad, on the other hand, was the most fearless man I've ever known. The invariably daunting situations and people I've witnessed him encounter were never enough to threaten his ability to make decisions. His whole rationale was defined by never doubting himself and never backing down, despite the consequences. He was determined to prevent every slight from breaking his psyche. He refused to show any weakness to his enemies because he recognized that those disadvantages would be used against him. He was, in every sense of the word, a warrior. I truly felt secure knowing that he was there protecting our family. We relied on him to remain calm, comforting, and a source of stability for all of us. The day that he died was one of the most devastating losses I would ever encounter.

Even with the best upbringing, I was born with this unique ability to question myself and the world around me. Left unmanaged, this quality could either become my greatest strength or my most damning weakness. The intention here is to tread backwards into my past where uncertainty, pain, and fear had been acquired and also reinforced by traumatic experience. I believe now my true purpose is to harness my worst characteristics into larger skill sets that will serve me well in the future.

When I became mentally strong enough, I employed this unique perspective to conquer my greatest psychological wounds. Only then was I able to stand out of my own way. I have come face to face with my worst nightmares and managed to rise back up from a defeated mindset. Most others would wake up to realize they were just dreaming, thinking nothing of it.

And maybe you too can learn to do the same, but only if you are willing to acknowledge your fear-related imperfections and use them to your advantage. It is critical to be honest in order to change. You can only deceive yourself so long before the truth begins to break through the cracks in the surface.

FACE INVISIBLE FEARS

I have been frightened by so many things, and for so long have been rendered unable to recognize where it all originates from. I had to detail those moments that made me shut down and not want to speak. So, I am vowing to process what had been unidentifiable. For years, I have suffered with mood changes, deep depressions, and never could understand why it was so hard to be happy. I hid my emotions and never spoke about what was bothering me. It came to the point where so many issues were compounded by trauma, that I even failed to recognize the origin.

In the process of re-constructing this detailed account of my experiences, I acquired a sense of perspective. I knew that if I targeted the root of my pain and recurring fears, I'd have the chance to be free of them. To live an unfettered existence would be the ultimate goal, but I had to endure this process until it no longer haunted me. And I refused to give up until I was at peace. The words I write will come to an end, but this journey will continue.

MY FIRST TEA PARTY

I have long suffered from post-traumatic stress disorder (PTSD) and anxiety due to traumatic experience. My first interaction with intense panic took place on my first play date when I was five years old. I eagerly agreed to go out with the red haired, green-eyed monster from preschool. Prior to that day, I found it suspicious that the popular girl in school wanted to hang out with me. I was far from being cool, being an introvert that proudly sported my oversized glasses. That should have been my first clue that something wasn't right.

At the start of the day, she and I went to McDonald's fast-food restaurant, ordering happy meals with those miniature princess toys at the bottom of the box. Shortly after, we arrived at her house. We pranced around chasing each other for a while, then reenacted a make-believe tea party with Barbies. I remember how much I had fun because it was the first time I had played with someone other than myself. I was delighted by the mutual laughter and enjoyment.

In the middle of the tea party, we were finding new outfits for the dolls and the girl wanted to show me her closet. She opened the double doors with small white wooden panels. I turned around to look, and she aggressively pushed me inside, locking the door.

I thought it was a joke at first and was even giggling. As each second stretched slowly into minutes, I snapped like a rubber band with too much tension. I knew I had been trapped in there for a long time because my body was drenched in sweat. I begged, screamed, and even pleaded for my friend to let me out. I could hear her mother's voice echoing in the background. I was certain that her mom heard me screaming for my life, but to my amazement, she did nothing. After a while, I was sure they invited to their home just so that they could torture me.

I was screaming so long for help that I lost my voice. My mouth continued the motions of speech, but nothing audible could surface. The smell of old shoes and mildew invaded my nasal cavity as my hands began to tremble from banging forcefully on the closet door. The fight in me had eventually dwindled down to an intermittent tap until my hands dropped entirely. My hands were red and now began to bruise, along with my delicate ego. I was a fool for thinking I could be best friends with the popular girl in school.

My sweaty hair stuck to the back of my neck as adrenaline coursed through my bulging veins. As my body heat began to cool, complete mental and physical exhaustion set in.

I don't even remember why, but she finally opened the door. Maybe it was her guilt, but I don't think so. I am almost certain she consumed a large dose of satisfaction from torturing me. It was as if hurting me was the drug she needed to get her fix. Once she got high, the intention was to dispose of the evidence using her mother. That's the only reason she opened the door.

I busted out of her room searching for answers. Oddly enough, her mother was standing in the corridor directly adjacent to Gillan's bedroom door. I tried to explain what her daughter just had done to me. But with a deluded peachy demeanor, she glared at me with amusement while I spoke. It was clear her goal was to convince me that I was being crazy. The intonation of her voice explained it all, despite the "my daughter could never do such a thing" defense. It was my belief that this woman knew exactly what her daughter was up to. She even guarded the bedroom door just to prevent interruption of her child's devious behavior. Her daughter, at the age of five, was becoming a monster because she was the spawn of one.

When my mom finally arrived to pick me up, I couldn't speak for hours. This streak of silence lasted for days. I couldn't speak because my mind was unable to make sense of the pain. I trusted an adult to take care of me, and she was an accomplice to her daughter's actions. It was beyond words to describe how someone could break the universal moral code underlying friendship and responsible parenting, just to hurt a child. I never understood the concept of evil until I looked the devil straight in the eye. With pleasure, they inflicted wounds deeper than the Band-Aid of love. I was an angel with broken wings; afraid to use my mangled parts to fly.

That was the first time my powerful voice could be muted. There were no words to express the kind of help I needed. Nothing could change what they did to me. I was so trusting. I failed to understand that no one would come to save me. The damage was done. The girl that went in the closet that day was not the same one who came out.

With my entrance into tight spaces and just closing my eyes for bed, I absorbed panic from my memories of that play date. Each time this memory interacted with me; I felt a surge of anxiety coursing through my blood. This was the first time I experienced flashbacks. I couldn't quite conceptualize the impact they had on me. I just knew I became triggered by certain moments and panic would take over my body until I lost control of my own sense of reason. With each flashback, I would become farther from the person I could identify in the mirror. And that's because I no longer had power over myself, instead I was under the control of that girl and the pain she left me with.

CONFRONTING THE DISTRUSTING ME

Over the years, I have recognized that this experience still haunts me. When I met someone with good intentions for the first time, I automatically questioned them. I was certain I would be disappointed. On the other hand, I understood that I could be wrong to assume a negative outcome. I knew I should not discount anyone prior to giving them a chance. It didn't help that the bullies from preschool to middle school had a target on my back. It was as if they could detect I was shy, vulnerable, insecure, and had low self-esteem.

During elementary school years, I had rocks thrown at my face, my hair pulled, and was called ugly. I even had friends for a few hours, who decided that their loyalty belonged somewhere else by the end of the school day. I think that had to do with the fact that I reached a breaking point. I began to explode internally. The next person in school who attempted to mess with me got what they deserved- the payback beat down. I was finally sticking up for myself and protecting my mental health. I was not going to make any compromises.

Even when I didn't want to, I provided new friends with the opportunity to become part of my life. Around the age of 12, I opened up and gave more chances, but with tight parameters. I didn't go out alone with them anywhere, didn't share my secrets, and definitely did not sleep over. The fate of a friendship depended on the level of hurt inflicted upon me. Once I was betrayed beyond repair, I cut friends from my life. Looking back, the strange headaches and stomach pains began to make sense. I noticed the stress from those situations had manifested as psychosomatic symptoms.

Much school therapy was required to acknowledge my negative thoughts regarding interactions with others. Due to the intense degree of bullying I had been the victim of, I developed immense distrust in others. I always thought I had a target on my back. I realized that the issue was not their behavior, or even what they might do to hurt me, it was my expectations. I set myself up to be disappointed by believing that friends are supposed to be honest and genuine one hundred percent of the time.

I concluded that most of my issues stemmed from my frigid expectations. How I set the standards for building trust is what mattered most. It would be beneficial to ask for small displays of accountability prior to requiring large duties to be fulfilled. Because I was quick to dismiss or eliminate others, I may have been culpable for failed relationships. The second mistake I made was labeling individuals as friends that didn't earn the title. As a consequence, my deep level of disappointment led to eliminating people from my life early on.

EXPANDING SOCIAL NETWORKS

From looking back at this time in my life, I have discovered the true value of making interpersonal connections. I can see all the meaningful friendships and work relationships that have had an immense impact on me. I am grateful to those who encouraged me to become more than I thought I could be. Those mentors along the way are the true heroes. In this story, their lessons become clear, based on the advice I provide. They reminded me to believe in myself again, and for that, I am so grateful. Because of the quality of those connections, I didn't need a thousand friends.

I am grateful for this period in my life because I learned

how to navigate interpersonal relationships. The following are some of the key changes I have made, which have made a drastic difference in the way I interact with others.

1. Portray yourself in a positive manner:

When I remained open-minded, honest, positive, and walked around with my head up, my energy was received as positive. If I made it obvious that I trusted no one, I received hostility from others. Displaying vulnerability made me a target for those looking to dominate with their power and control. My problematic behavior became abundantly clear when I witnessed individuals walking around avoiding eye contact, being entirely uncertain of themselves. I realized that lacking faith and confidence in myself caused me to be considered weak. Simply by walking with my head down and speaking to people without looking at them, my intentions were questioned. As soon as I began to change my vocal tone, increased eye contact, and believed in myself, my interpersonal relationships started to change. Those around me were able to witness my spirit blossom magnetically, and that's the kind of friend they wanted in their corner.

2. Trust is earned, not given:

The greatest lesson was that there were negative consequences when I fully trusted someone before knowing anything about them. I would even believe their words would always match their actions. From that time, I know that trust must be earned, not given. Years after that play date, I learned more about the person I needed to become to prevent my heart from being broken. I no longer felt obligated to provide full trust without good reason. Day by day and moment by moment, there are opportunities to validate words and behavior. If a person's behavior demonstrates that they are not being truthful, trust that. This will be your sign that they have ulterior motives.

3. Stand up for yourself in a constructive manner: When you are feeling insulted by someone you care about, it is necessary to make sure you defend yourself. By this, I do not mean respond with a physical attack. In actuality, you need to verbalize your emotions in a firm manner. Say how you feel and why it made you upset. Being firm allows the person to understand that it is not okay to hurt you again. Through this process, the person will realize what it was that made their words or actions unnecessarily harsh.

4. Set boundaries for respect and reinforce them: Boundaries require making a set of rules that define what is acceptable versus what isn't. In a friendship there are expectations and standards that you hold your friend to. For example, you expect your friend to not speak bad about you to others or steal your partner. If you make these rules clear from the beginning, it prevents them from unintentionally causing a rift between you. Secondly, there needs to be consequences for violating the boundaries such as loss of friendship or having a conversation about it. Otherwise, you will quickly become a doormat to be taken advantage of. Being in this position before, it negatively affected my emotions.

5. Desensitize yourself to social interaction:
While trying to repair my socialization issues, I learned that it is important to not allow the past experiences prevent you from trying again. Not every person is out to hurt you. Taking this into consideration, I made sure to give this a try. I did not find it fun to panic in a crowded room. So, one day, I sat down at a full table in the dining room at school and introduced myself to the people sitting down. After meeting them, it was like my fear went away. They were all respectful to me and I definitely appreciated that since I was a complete stranger. Taking the time to randomly introduce myself in public places, I learned how to better communicate with others. Best of all, I was no longer afraid to put myself out there for criticism. Not everyone would like me, but that should not stop me from trying to make new friends.

6. Those that hurt you are hurting too:
When reflecting on the times that friends have lashed out at me in the past, I urged myself to take their perspective.

So I imagined what it would be like to live in their shoes. Doing so led to a major epiphany. I realized that those who seek to hurt me are looking for a way to dispose of their own pain. This may be coming from their family life, upbringing, or a negative environment. Maybe they were involved in traumatic experiences as well. I cannot be sure. But what I do know is that you cannot hold onto pain forever because it will cause you to explode on others. This is why it is necessary to find healthy ways to cope with our own emotions.

References

Marie Curie Quotes. (n.d.).
https://www.brainyquote.com/quotes/marie_curie_389010

2

THE SUPPOSITION OF LOSS

> *"No one ever told me that grief felt like fear"*
>
> — *C. S. LEWIS*

When I was young, I failed to comprehend the finality of death. I reasoned that whoever was plagued with illness would somehow resurrect if I just prayed hard enough. In some strange way, I knew this couldn't actually be possible. But I always hoped it would be. I believed in miracles.

During the early 2000s, I encountered my first experience with death. The sound of the news echoed in ripples, and with each crash to my heart, I endured another jolting dose of pain. He was my Uncle. He was best described by his casual and delightful demeanor, wide green eyes on a tall, thin body frame. Present at many of our family functions and birthdays, he was a great friend and support system to my parents. He had an outgoing personality and always brought a smile to the room he entered.

But here's the thing, he wasn't actually my real uncle. He was so close to our family that we considered him as such. Unbeknownst to all of us, he secretly suffered from liver cirrhosis as a consequence of his lifestyle choices. Because this happened with no warning signs, family and friends were stunned. At first, I was uncertain how to react upon receiving the news. I failed to grasp that this meant I would no longer see him. I was sad when my mother explained that he was gone for good and would not be returning. As she explained to me, the purpose of a funeral service was to say our last goodbyes and celebrate life. Tears of pain and discussion of past memories are typical occurrences. But even this explanation did not suffice for the emotions that were invoked within me that day.

The day of the service, I struggled to get ready. This was my first time, but my mom said that when we lament, we wear dark clothes. The attire signifies a state of mourning. As we pulled up, we could see quite a few family members smoking outside with a deep grimace on their faces, which was enhanced by granulations in the darkness of night. We followed the crowd by finding other relatives to exchange sentiments with. Shortly after, we went through the front entrance into the parlor doors, tiptoeing to the back of the service. Standing in the back of the funeral home, I grieved quietly. There was a somber silence that brought chills along my body in waves. I walked hesitantly towards the open casket with my head held down, envisioning my last words to him. He was visibly bluish and brown colored, but this was camouflaged by make-up. When I touched his arm, it was ice cold. It was at that moment I realized that death refers to the loss of the physical body, where the inner spirit becomes released from its capsule. The only thing that remains is an empty vessel for us to believe they are with us for just one second, so we can have closure. But being so young, this was my first time being presented with the concept of finality, so I was questioning this outcome as permanent.

Towards the end of the service, various family members gathered at the front altar to reminisce about their love for him. I desperately wanted to say something, but I was only 11 years old, with no experience in public speaking. I trembled at the thought of choking on my words and the embarrassment that would ensue. I thought to myself, that no one cared to hear my thoughts anyway. As I stood in the back of the room, I heard muffled voices of the mourning crowd above the speech I was making in my head for him. Each time the priest at the front asked if anyone wanted to speak, I hesitated. I trembled like a faulty engine from the thought of exposing my vulnerable emotions. A sense of nagging guilt plagued me for years after failing to express my love and appreciation for him. It was hurtful, holding back those words for decades; they played on a loop in my mind.

THE ORANGE STRIPED KITTEN

While recuperating from my uncle's loss, I was close to encountering another one. I remember it was a sunny day and the rays were warming the surface of my skin. My brother and I were riding our bikes on the streets of our Westfield home when we noticed an orange striped kitten. He alerted me to its presence and I was immediately awestruck. The kitten was curious and incredibly fluffy, with bright yellow stunning eyes. He began to prance over to us with his tail high in the air as we looked on in amazement. We had never witnessed such beauty in a small creature. It was not long before my brother lured the kitten over into his arms. Once we had him in our possession, we were determined to bring him home. The next step involved manipulating mom into allowing us to keep him. My brother and I had a quick huddle to discuss how we could gently coerce mom into saying "yes."

I decided that my brother would be more convincing. He was the feline lover, above all other animals. And he was in fact, the first-born son, with more pull on my mothers' emotions. There was no denying that he was the favorite, even after I came along. He had the perfect mocha colored skin, sparkling white teeth, and all the charm that could go with it. Moreso, he had this ability to apply the pressure of intense guilt to get his way. I hate to say it, but it worked. It always has. When it comes to me, yes, I've always been more independent. I could have cried, and still would not have received the same level of attention.

On our short journey back to the house, we ran into my mother outside. My brother embraced the kitten in his arms with so much excitement to show off our new discovery to mom. It was then I noticed an apparent shift in her demeanor. I suspect that it was slight anger mixed with confusion. I was thinking there was no way she would say yes. Besides, my mother usually was firm in her sticking to her decisions. Anticipation of her reaction caused my heart to flutter and my shirt to stick to my sweat-drenched chest.

As she pivoted towards us, her eyes widened. If any of you were to meet her, you would know this is her signature facial expression for all matters serious, dramatic, ridiculous, and humorous. Before she was able to utter one word, my brother's ability to manipulate her emotions was already at work. I looked on in amazement as his tactics were strategic and effective on my mother.

He stretched out his arms and presented the kitten as if it were on display in an animal abuse commercial. Much more easily than I could have accomplished, he made his case. He told her the baby was a cute, starved, neglected bag of bones in desperate need for love. Unable to reject his valid argument, she hesitantly agreed that we could keep the cat, so long as it did not have any diseases. In that moment, I just knew she had also recognized the beauty in this creature. She just could not say no.

The first few nights we worked on picking a name, going back and forth we decided on Leighlah, based on the popular song. That was also because we did not truly know if the cat was female or male until he further developed. The name was fitting, I had to admit, this lovely feline had us wrapped around his paw. This became evident by the way we catered to his every need. Over the next few days, we nursed the kitten back to health. It wasn't long before we began to build a bond so strong that we worshiped the ground on which Leighlah pranced. In fact, we relished in our playtime with him so much that we often willingly neglected our schoolwork.

To be honest, Leighlah was considered to be the 5th member of our family. It was not as though I took him for granted. My family and I gave all the love we had. But to our surprise, he was starting to show signs of sickness. I never have envisioned that my worst nightmare would come to fruition even after a visit to the vet. But it happened. My first connection with an animal was being threatened by an outside source that I was entirely unaware of at the time.

One day he was playing on his tree house while I was doing homework at the kitchen table. I looked over prompted by a curious noise; gurgling mixed with gasps for air. I didn't know how to make sense of this. Immediately jumped up from my seat and walked towards him. Just before I could reach out my hand to stop it, he fell abruptly off the tree house. He laid on the floor gasping for air with all four paws sticking straight out as if he were paralyzed. I was devastated. I had never seen this before and I did not know what to do. So I picked him up and held him just doing my best to comfort my baby. As he laid in my arms, time stood still. I just remember the sound of his every breath echoing throughout my body. I continued to hold him until my mom arrived to help.

Scared as we could be, my mom did the honorable thing and held Leighla all night while he slept. He was struggling to hold on to the last bit of life left in him. He lost control of his bowels and motor functions. And still my mom provided him with a sense of dignity by not worrying about being covered in urine so that his last night with her could remain as normal as possible. I looked up to my mom for showing such compassion towards our suffering cat. I honored her because she cared for him just as she would me or my brother. She became a role-model for how to treat animals ethically. I truly learned to regard pets as sentient beings capable of experiencing love and pain. After the rough night of coddling our orange kitty, she rushed him to the animal hospital first thing in the morning.

The veterinarians performed a series of tests and bloodwork. After a couple of hours, my brother, mom and I were informed that he had Leukemia. The doctors explained that this was a lethal form of blood cancer. In other words, there was nothing that could be done to save him. To end Leighla's suffering, it was recommended that we euthanize him. For me, this evoked the instant need to vomit. I ran outside for some air to stop suffocating from the devastating news. My mom remained inside saying goodbye to our beloved baby. I just did not have the courage to stand by watching the life drift from his little body. I believed that all the cries in the world would not be powerful enough to save me from this kind of heartache.

Looking back, it would not be fair to say that I was just weak in nature. But I was feeling defeated because I lacked enough life experience to know whether or not what I was doing was right. Upon reflection of this decision as an adult, I do believe my mom was justified in her reasoning for putting him down. Our pet was suffering from a serious illness that takes the lives of millions of humans daily, so to draw out his torture would have been cruel to say the least.

I left that clinic that day with regret for being unable to say goodbye, like the death of Uncle. I always hoped I would wake up and realize it was all a bad dream. From this moment forward, I began to fear death and the effect its permanence had on me.

This feeling became worse as I encountered more death, like my Aunt (mom's sister) who passed on from a rare autoimmune disease known as Scleroderma. I also never had the chance to say my parting words since her death came abruptly.

Just when I thought things were going to be safe, Hurricane Irene forced us to evacuate our seaside home. We ended up going to our family's house up north Jersey to get away from the island. During that time, my beloved grandmother was becoming sicker from diabetes, kidney disease, and an ongoing heart condition.

As she approached her final days, I was informed by one of my aunts that she was nearing the end. I dropped whatever I was doing and ran to her bedside. Although I was not sure if it would be the last moment, I treated it as such. I grabbed her hands, looked her in the eyes, and told her I loved her. Being able to do this provided me with relief, but was also incredibly hurtful to accept. After receiving the call around 3 am, this sickness infected my soul, a deep distaste rotted in the pit of my stomach. This was because I was forced to adjust to a new life without her there. For me, that was hard to accept since I was so close with her over the years.

This was the third service I had attended. Despite missing my grandmother so much, I was able to rejoice and celebrate her life by speaking at the front podium. Even more special were the moments I shared with my father. I could feel that he was proud of me for speaking for the family. As hard as it was, I was proud that I finally had the courage to do it.

MY PATERNAL GRANDFATHER

To rub salt in my exposed wounds, I lost my paternal grandfather maybe a year or two later. Because of the other deaths I have encountered, the thought of dealing with another one led to intense physical and emotional reactions. The last day of my grandfather's life was tortuous; he suffered from Emphysema and COPD, conditions related to the health hazards of his job and smoking.

We initially received the news of his rapid decline after receiving a phone call from his wife. She told us that his lungs were shutting down due to fluid accumulation. In other words, he was drowning in his own fluid. After receiving that call, I swear my mother did 90 mph on the parkway to get to Bergen County, New Jersey, which is two hours north of Seaside Park. During the drive, I witnessed my father silently sobbing with his head down, sipping his beer to numb the pain. At that moment, who could blame him for wanting to drink. No one wants to lose a parent, even though we all know it's inevitable.

After arriving at the nursing home, my father and I

approached the room down the hall to the left. We took a look at the person in the bed, and he was far from appearing like the man we knew. My dad took a hard look and walked back out. He refused to believe that it was his father. He looked so frail that he was no longer recognizable as the man we knew. He was barely 100 pounds and looked like a shell of a human being. I looked on in sadness as each attempt to draw in oxygen was followed by shallow gurgling breaths. I never saw my father cry in that way until that moment. It ripped my heart into a million pieces. I felt his pain, plus that of my own. I couldn't bear to see my father suffer. It ate away at my soul.

As I looked on, I realized that my grandfather's soul was already gone but his empty vessel remained. I said my goodbyes hoping he would hear them from the other side, all the while comforting my father as much as possible. On our way back home, we received a call that he had passed.

A LOSS I STRUGGLED TO ACCEPT

As it turns out, I would have to say goodbye to another blood relative only 11 months later. This is after my grandfather's passing in January of my senior year at Rutgers University. As I was about to graduate, I received the news that I was missing credits for graduation. This was because the department changed the degree requirements without informing me. I initially planned on taking summer classes to resolve this matter, but none of the classes I needed were being offered. So I went back to classes in the fall.

After moving back on campus, I decided to visit my family. I went home around the time of my birthday in early October. My father said Charlie, our dog, could use another friend, so my mom and I looked, not realizing that he knew he was dying. We just didn't recognize his progressing illness because we were so happy about getting another dog. So, we went to adopt a cute puppy named Lucy. After we came back with her, my father was happy but not concerned that she was being aggressive towards his baby Charlie. Within days after the adoption, I noticed my father was sleeping a lot. Because he sat with no lamp on, while watching his TV, we didn't even notice the signs of serious liver failure. He became increasingly lethargic as time went on. I came to realize that he was waking up almost as if he didn't know where he was. Being that out of touch with reality, I noticed he was speaking about events that weren't really happening. For example, he would believe there were people there trying to attack him, or not remember that I was there. That weekend in particular was my birthday and I tried to wake him up to remind him. When he opened his eyes, I asked him if he would spend my birthday with me. But he looked at me as if I weren't there. Then, he rolled back over and went back to sleep. I immediately told my mom something was wrong. He was showing signs of some kind of memory impairment, which made me concerned. At the time, I was not an expert on these matters, but I knew what was normal and what was not. I do not enjoy celebrating my birthday because of this moment. It deeply saddened me to realize that my dad was beginning to forget me.

After describing his behavior to my mother, she immediately left her room and went to turn the light on to look at him. He sat up and my mom asked him if he was okay. While checking on him she could see something appeared to be seriously wrong - his skin looked kind of greyish. Because of this, her concerns grew. My mom told him she was going to take him to the hospital for further checking. It wasn't until we started out the door, going down the steps, we could see the jaundice in his scalp and in the whites in his eyes. From that point on, all of us were in deep panic but at the same time we tried to remain calm. With a childlike innocence, he agreed to go to the hospital for further testing. When we got him there, he was dizzy and unable to walk without assistance just going down the steps. After admitting him through the emergency room, they performed a series of tests on him to evaluate his bloodwork, brain, liver, and kidney functions. After a battery of tests, I was terrified to find out what the results would be. I had a feeling the results wouldn't be good. I was right.

The thought of losing my dad became a concern that kept me in emotional distress. It was no longer a run of the mill worry. I began to have terrible dreams, panic, cold sweats, and hyperventilation on the regular basis.

Only a week into his hospital stay, my mom received a phone call from the team of doctors. They informed her that he had fluid accumulation in his brain because his liver was shutting down. Since his health issues were irreversible, he could not be resuscitated. For me, this was hard to accept. I maintained hope that he could be saved until the last moment. The doctors told us my dad would be on the liver transplant list, but the chances of receiving one would be slim to none.

Over the next few days, he became increasingly incoherent. I would leave the room for several minutes and return to find out his memory reset to another place in time. One time, I went to the bathroom and upon returning, discovered he failed to remember my entire visit. This is one of the reasons I have suffered for years. It broke my heart to know that our past was no longer relevant; our father-daughter bond was slipping away.

During his hospital stay, I did my best to remain positive while the nurses pumped him with morphine and corticosteroids to jumpstart his liver and kidney function. Since he was in the process of dying, they offered to get him into a long-term rehabilitation facility. Immediately following the transfer to the rehab, his vital signs were slightly improved. This gave us all reason to believe that there could be hope. Being naive, I believed that this is something he could recover from. In my eyes, he was the strongest man I ever knew. I refused to accept that he couldn't beat this.

During our visits we would clean him up, bring him clean clothes, and provide him with dignity since he was uncomfortable with those nurses changing him. By this point, he was looking just like my grandfather. It had only been eleven months since his father died. But the similarities between them were apparent. My dad was frail like his father. He was a bag of skin on bones. I looked heavy at 100 pounds in comparison.

Watching him deteriorate started to break me down over the final days. All of us were exhausted from going back and forth from the hospital. But staying home was not an option. When you love someone that much, nothing will stop you from seeing them. I didn't care if I was dead tired and unable to walk straight. I made it my business to be there, even if that meant being broke and starving for days. There were several occasions where we struggled as a family to travel back and forth with so little money. On Thanksgiving Day, we were down to our last dollar on our way to visit him. While driving down the highway, we ran out of gas. Feeling defeated, mom pulled over. Just as she put her hazards on and looked in the rearview mirror, it was as if an angel pulled up right behind us. It was a retired officer who saw us. So he pulled over and immediately came up to my mom's car window and asked if we needed help. She explained to him what was going on. He took her to get gas and within 10 minutes we were back on our way. We were devastated because we didn't want to break our promise to have Thanksgiving dinner together.

Still to this day, I believe that this was a miracle. No one had ever shown our family an act of kindness such as this. I will be forever in debt to this person for allowing me to have this last holiday with my father. If you ever read this, I am grateful from the bottom of my heart.

After our dinner together, my mom and I took my father out into the rehab courtyard to get some air. He loved the food, feeling stable for the first time in weeks, and enjoyed his trip outdoors. That night my mother, brother, and I went home with smiles on our faces. We felt joy because my father seemed at peace for at least one day during his torturous battle against stage four liver failure. For those last twenty-four to forty-eight hours, his vitals appeared to be dramatically improved in comparison to his symptoms. Reflecting on this now, it was most likely the calm before the storm.

Later that night after we left, my father called and asked why we did not show up that day. He kept leaving his room and getting agitated because he couldn't remember us being there. He continued to sneak out until they had to have a guard watch his door. My dad was not the kind of man to be afraid of anything. So, I know this must be his illness taking over and making his brain believe falsehoods that threatened his psychological stability. During the course of that next day, he was transferred back through the emergency room and re-admitted into the Intensive Care Unit (ICU). At this time, it was almost my brother's birthday, December 1st.

As the 29th progressed, I noticed that my dad was wrestling between two worlds - the living and the dead. From this point, he was in a lot of physical pain and under a lot of sedation. His bare and boney legs were kicking around the bedsheets. It was as if he were trying to fight to get up and try. The father I knew would not allow this illness to defeat him. I knew deep down that he wanted to come home and be with our family.

The hospital staff had also noticed he was thrashing around the bed and so, they tried to restrain him. We would not allow that to happen. My mother and I did not believe it was fair to make someone feel like a prisoner in their final moments. During this time, they were also actively changing him because he had been losing blood through his urine and excrement. It looked like he was being amputated in front of me. Those images were difficult to erase or even subdue. During one particular time of being changed, my brother and I were standing in the hallway. I could hear his screams echoing throughout the whole floor of the hospital. I knew he was in a lot of pain, but I was awestruck at this determination to try and stay alive for my mom, brother, and I. Regardless of the memory loss, he knew my brother's birthday and Christmas were coming. I believed that he did not want to break our hearts.

After a few hours standing in the hospital room, I saw his blood pressure slowly dropping. At first, we all thought it was returning to normal. That is because it was finally in the normal range after being consistently high. When it reached the point of no return, I felt my lungs cave in and I dropped to my knees because it was finally becoming real that this would probably be my last night with him. The nurses offered him morphine drops to alleviate his unbearable levels of pain. However, the drawback was that it would instantly stop his breathing. Maybe it's selfish of me, but I asked that she didn't give him any more sedation since I wanted him to hear me talking to him.

As much as it hurt me, I had to help him end this pain. My mom realized it was no longer fair for us to put so much pressure on him to survive. My mom asked us to say our goodbyes so she could have her private time with him. I went over to his bedside and grabbed onto his hand tightly. I whispered in his ear that it was okay to go to the other side., I reminded him that I was there and to not be afraid. I tried to ease his guilt about leaving us in the physical world.

After speaking to my dad for a few minutes, he had a moment of clarity. My heart almost stopped when he opened his eyes to verbally acknowledge my presence. It was then that I told him that it is okay to go. That is the greatest gift I could have received in a devastating situation. I am proud of him for working the program and fighting against all odds to get better. Despite my ability to say the right things, my heart felt like it was being crushed into a million pieces. There are no words to describe the agony I endured.

Saying goodbye to my father was the most painful moment of my life. I knew that putting myself back together would be a challenge. After riding on this roller coaster for hours, the nurses came to the room. They told us that the process of "going" could take minutes, hours, or days. They would call us if his condition changed. Because we were all so emotionally drained, we took the ride home. It seemed okay to leave since we were only 15 minutes from the hospital.

When we got back to our apartment, we all fell asleep from exhaustion. Only a few minutes into my rest, I was awoken by the call that made my world stand still. My mom picked up the phone and her facial expression just said it all. He was gone.

I just felt as though my soul was ripped out of my body. My spirit was flooded by disappointment and guilt for not being able to save him. My years-long battle to cure him was over. His disease won. It was something that I had to accept, but I didn't want to. Even in those moments right after he was gone, I did not want to believe it was true. In order to truly accept it, I had to see him one last time. So, we returned to the hospital to take care of the after-death arrangements and say my final words.

When we arrived at his room, I noticed that the nurses cleaned up all the blood that was draining from his body externally. I was grateful that the nurse took the time to give him back his dignity in those last moments.

I remember my mom taking the chance to say her last words to him alone. It took me some time to muster up the courage to walk back in that room knowing that he was gone. I could not comprehend it was real, I didn't want to believe I would be forced to live the rest of my life with a part of me missing. After panicking in the hallway, hyper-ventilating for quite some time, I reminded myself that this was my last chance to say goodbye. As I approached his bedside, my head was pounding, my eyes were swollen, and my heart was jumping through my chest.

I was in such shock that I actually believed he was still breathing. My eyes kept playing tricks on me. Maybe it was all a bad dream. I prayed that I would wake up the next day and my world would be back to normal. But it wasn't. After saying my last words, I felt like a part of my soul had been ripped out of my chest. I had no energy left from crying. My dad truly meant the world to me. I loved him regardless of his struggle with addiction. I hope he knew that I loved him unconditionally and that I no longer blamed him for being an alcoholic.

During this moment, my brother was in immense shock, since it had now been the morning of his birthday. As a result, he was not experiencing the same emotional breakdown that I was. He was holding me in the hallway as I sobbed uncontrollably. And I told him he should walk in there, otherwise forever feel guilty for saying nothing. So, he followed my advice and said his piece.

By this point, we decided to go home because we were functioning on autopilot from deep exhaustion. I was still shocked at how composed my brother was compared to my mother and I. As we approached the hospital's exit his demeanor changed. He dropped to his knees and went into a full meltdown, releasing this visceral noise that came from his gut and radiated throughout the hospital lobby. My mom and I held onto him giving him all of our strength and love. I knew lifting his spirits would require more than just my mom and I picking him up from the floor that night.

Following this night, my brother laid down in bed and didn't move for seven days. Even worse, he did not say one word to us the whole time. It was as if his pain led to a full mind and body paralysis. I have never seen my brother in this condition before. It truly bothered me that I could not take away his suffering. To make matters worse, we both developed pneumonia. After a few days, Mom and I got up to plan a small memorial service, while he remained in bed.

This loss was much different than those before it. My

sense of positivity, optimism, and joy was sucked from my spirit. Simple tasks were taxing. Even speaking to people in the outside world made me panic. From my previous experience with loss, it is difficult for someone else to understand your feelings. This is because your life experiences are generally unparalleled to others. No one has the right to define how long your grieving process should be.

For myself in particular, I experienced a rough transition back into my normal life. I believe that my level of bereavement worsened over time because of the complicated past with my father. There were so many memories and words left unfinished. I spent months suffering through the graphic images of him bleeding to death, and months of disturbing hallucinations. What hurt most was that he struggled to remember my existence. Those thoughts made my head spin until I was entirely consumed. I couldn't eat, sleep, or live anymore. The problem was that no immediate resolution exists for this kind of psychological torment. These kinds of complicated losses are not easy to overcome.

Because of sleep disturbances and active flashbacks became so unbearable. I turned to alcohol and drugs. This was the only way I felt able to disconnect from the memories long enough to rest. During that time, the only people who understood me were my family. They had endured the same moments with me and I knew it also impacted them negatively. It made me angry when people would expect me to be better overnight. As a result, I isolated myself from the rest of the world. This fearful behavior was only reinforced by harsh and judgmental social interactions. People expected me to just get over it, or assumed that because a few weeks had passed, I would go back to my usual radiant self. Little did they know, they were so wrong. It got so bad that it actually pained me to communicate about any aspect of my life to anyone.

Roughly 6 months had passed, and I realized that I needed to clear my head and restart my mind. I decided to stop drinking and using drugs recreationally so that I could be in a more coherent state of mind to face my inner demons. I thought if I learned about my symptoms, I would understand them better. And in doing so, I believed that I would experience some healing.

I was uncertain about how this would help me, but I had this underlying sense of faith. Besides what could I lose? I decided to do some research on prolonged or complicated grief to see if there was anything I could do to jumpstart my recovery. I suspected that understanding the twists and turns of bereavement would be crucial for me to experience drastic psychological improvements.

THE BEREAVEMENT PROCESS

Most individuals in their lifetime mourn the loss of a loved one. Regardless of the circumstances surrounding death, it can be life changing. That devastation may initiate a cycle of grief with no clear end or beginning. For those who have not endured death, this concept may seem foreign. Based on the Hospice Foundation of America, grief is described as a reaction to loss, such as deep sorrow or pain (HPA, 2018). Yet this definition just barely scratches the surface of what some people actually endure in the months and years following death. As more research is conducted, it becomes clear that grief affects each individual differently (Neimeyer, 2005).

As initially proposed by Elisabeth Kubler-Ross in her 1969 book entitled *Death and Dying*, grief can include, but is not limited to Denial, Anger, Depression, Bargaining, and Acceptance. Collectively, these stages are known as the bereavement period. When enduring denial, there is marked difficulty coping and a refusal to believe the finality of death. This stems from being unable to address the magnitude of pain that comes with acceptance. In this stage, individuals actively deny the reality of loss by employing distractions. For example, you will see someone burying themselves in work to prevent subconscious feelings of sadness from emerging.

In comparison to denial, anger manifests itself in various forms. For example, unresolved matters with the person who has died can lead to a sense of resentment and blame. In the midst of anger, friendships and family relationships can be destroyed by irrational thoughts such as

"Why did you have to enable your sister's drinking? It's your fault that she died." In fact, feelings of anger during mourning may lead to maladaptive coping strategies such as excessive drug use, partying, and even isolation. The emotional complexities within this stage are endless, but it is imperative to become aware of these issues in order to heal properly. Being educated about the bereavement process also prevents any undue stigma.

Bargaining becomes evident when the victim pleads for the return of their loved one by negotiating to have them back. Oftentimes you will hear someone saying: "I would trade anything in the world just to have my mother back, even if it is just for one second." This stage is also where feelings of guilt creep in. People may blame themselves for things they didn't say or do to improve the situation. That guilt propels the need to bargain or try to reiterate different scenarios in their minds that would have changed the outcome of death. This is one of the most difficult stages of grief to endure because this kind of thinking leads to sleep deprivation, depression, and unrelenting feelings of anger towards oneself.

The Stage of Acceptance comes into fruition when the individual who experienced loss is able to not only obtain a sense of closure, but also come to accept the reality of death. At this point, there is the ability to compartmentalize the loss as outside of one's own control and eliminate a sense of guilt, blame, or depression, because that person has been able to deal, rather than resorting to maladaptive coping strategies.

Although Kubler-Ross' work has provided great insight to support a generalized understanding of grief, research has displayed that 10% of all bereaved persons end up with complicated grief (Middleton et al., 1993 & Prigerson et al., 2009). In fact, for some individuals, bereavement can be much more complex than initially thought. Therefore, clinicians have worked to make diagnostic criteria that distinguishes complicated grief from recurring traumatic memories consistent with Post-Traumatic Stress Disorder (PTSD), and Major Depressive Disorder (MDD).

ACUTE GRIEF

According to Prigerson et al. (2009), acute grief commonly occurs within 6-12 months following the loss of a loved one. Common symptoms include recurrent and strong feelings of yearning, pangs of deep sadness or remorse (episodes of crying), steady and vivid thoughts and images of the deceased, a struggle to accept the reality of the death concurrent with feelings of anger. However, there may also be somatic symptoms (body sensations) such as uncontrollable sighing, digestive symptoms, loss of appetite, sleep disturbances, exhaustion and weakness, restlessness, and difficulty initiating or maintaining organized activities. There is also a sense of feeling disconnected from the world or other people, whereby the individual becomes indifferent and irritable with others. Grief becomes considered complicated when there is persistence of symptoms of acute grief. Furthermore, there is a presence of thoughts, feelings and behaviors reflecting distracting concerns about the circumstances surrounding death.

COMPLICATED VERSUS NON-COMPLICATED GRIEF

Complicated grief (CG) refers to prolonged, unabated grief where strong attachments to the deceased activate rewards systems that evoke yearning concurrent with pain when presented with stimuli regarding death (O'Connor et al., 2008). On the other hand, non-complicated grief (NCG) patients display the ability to experience brief pain and do not have prolonged yearning or reward activation in response to loss related stimuli (Horowitz, 2003). Earlier work on grief supports the framework for current classifications of NCG and CG by presenting a model of reunion versus detachment, whereby the loss of a loved one evokes either a strong desire to reunite, or an ability to accept the loss and move forward by detaching oneself from the outcome of death (Bowlby, 1979; 2018).

DSM-5 CRITERION FOR PERSISTENT COMPLEX BEREAVEMENT- RELATED DISORDER

The following are the current diagnostic features of complicated grief.

- The patient experienced the death of a loved one at least six months previously

At least ***one*** of the following symptoms has been present longer than expected, taking into account the person's social or cultural environment:

- Intense and persistent yearning for the deceased;
- Frequent preoccupation with the deceased;
- Intense feelings of emptiness or loneliness;
- Recurrent thoughts that life is meaningless or unfair without the deceased;
- A frequent urge to join the deceased in death.

At least ***two*** of the following symptoms have been recorded for at least one month:

- Feelings of disbelief or inability to accept the loss;
- Rumination about the circumstances or consequences of the death;

- Anger or bitterness about the death;
- Experiencing pain that the deceased suffered, or hearing/seeing the deceased;
- Trouble trusting or caring about others;
- Intense reactions to memories or reminders of the deceased;
- Avoidance of reminders of the deceased, or the opposite - seeking out reminders to feel close to the deceased.

Symptoms cause substantial distress for the sufferer or impact significantly on areas of functioning and cannot be attributed to other causes (Black & Grant, 2014).

CRITICISMS OF DSM-IV DIAGNOSTIC CRITERIA

According to an article by Paul A. Boelen (2016), there are several issues with the DSM-IV in regard to complicated grief. The primary concern with the proposed criteria for Persistent Complex Bereavement is over the characteristics required to yield a diagnosis. First, the DSM requires that at least one of the four core symptoms be present within a six-month time period. The issue with this is that these symptoms tend to coexist with degrees of severity which can become more problematic when all four symptoms are present. In other words, this means that there are many ways that these conditions can be satisfied while also remaining similar to other mental disorders. In this regard, it would be beneficial to have a more discrete and exclusive definition of complex, disturbed grief.

Having too much inclusion only leads to questions surrounding accuracy of the criteria. This makes it difficult to properly treat individuals suffering with this disorder. Being a survivor of grief, I began to wonder how I could develop coping mechanisms to deal with the multitude of symptoms I was facing. I know for a fact from experimenting with self-medicating via alcohol and drug use that these methods are entirely unsuccessful. Nothing cures the yearning better than using the source of the pain to alleviate your symptoms.

REWARD SYSTEM PROCESSING DURING CHRONIC DRUG USE

When drugs are introduced into a naive subject, this alters reward processing through the mesolimbic dopamine system. The normal behavioral response to natural rewards such as food, sex, and water become secondary as first time drug use becomes habitual. In other words, drugs hijack the brain, making these natural rewards or simple pleasures secondary (Koob, 2003; 2009).

NEUROBIOLOGICAL MECHANISMS OF GRIEF

Because love and attachments are neurobiologically similar to drug addiction, the absence of those bonds can elicit intense withdrawal symptoms that produce cravings (Burkett & Young, 2012). According to O'Connor & Colleagues (2008), the Nucleus accumbens (NAC) is a key structure responsible for reward signaling during drug-taking, social attachment, and maternal behavior via the mesolimbic dopamine (DA) system. Their research suggests that the NAC is activated in individuals with chronic grief. They also suspect that the NAC is responsible for invoking yearning during long term bereavement. This indicates that enduring grief may induce cravings for love via activation of these drug reward circuits.

GENETIC CHANGES IN REWARD SYSTEMS DURING CHRONIC DRUG USE AS A PREDICTOR FOR PROLONGED GRIEF

According to Nestler & Aghajanian (1997), chronic opiate use leads to a compensatory up-regulation of a secondary messenger known as Cyclic Adenosine Monophosphate (cAMP). This messenger leads to increases in adenylyl cyclase and cAMP dependent in the Protein Kinase A (PKA). Essentially, this is the biological effect of prolonged drug use. On the other hand, acute opiate exposure results in inhibition of the cAMP pathway. As Nestler and colleagues assert, up-regulation of this pathway is an indicator of increased physiological tolerance. In the absence of the opiate, the up-regulated pathway becomes fully functional and enhances the features of dependence and withdrawal.

When there is an absence of drugs after chronic use, this leads to intense craving and yearning. Because of the preliminary research, it may be possible that these neurochemical pathways undergo similar changes during late stages of grief. If researchers constructed a paradigm allowing for experimentation of control versus bereaved subjects, evaluating cAMP may serve as a useful measure.

NEW APPROACHES FOR AN OLD PROBLEM

Although research on the relationship between prolonged grief and genetics is in its infancy, biological changes within reward systems may be an underlying mechanism by which the primary symptoms of bereavement persist. Understanding the relationships between reward, genetics, and behavior is only one critical component required for advancements in treatment. Furthermore, it is necessary to acknowledge those enduring chronic grief during primary evaluations, in order to prompt focused research. In order to aid those suffering, there would need to be more specificity in the diagnostic criterion. In concordance with this, researchers can guide clinicians on bereavement, using similar strategies employed for treatment of chronic drug use. If feelings of yearning, wanting, and withdrawal can be adequately managed using similar techniques employed for preventing drug relapse, patients have a better chance at making improvements.

This proposed solution does not exclude the need for benefits provided by treatment of other comorbid conditions. In other words, other forms of therapy would serve as an adjunct to techniques used for absolving patients from long-term grief. We should hold steadfast in our work towards educating ourselves as friends, clinicians, and researchers, so that those fighting the battle against devastation have the opportunity to overcome it. From the clinical perspective, there are several strategies that are not often incorporated in the healing process.

TRANSITION FROM FEAR TO ACCEPTANCE: STEPS TOWARDS IMPROVEMENT

Taking a closer look at the series of devastating losses in my young life has led to several epiphanies. First, the magnitude of loss is proportional to the amount of love. I love my dad, grandfather, grandmother, Uncle, Aunt, and my cats. I believe that because I was attached securely with these people and animals, I was greatly impacted by their deaths.

The thought of becoming attached to any person or animal frightened me. Even considering the uncertainty around newfound love and loss made me nauseated and terrified. I just wanted to remain as superficially connected to others as possible. That fear even guided my motivations, decisions, and behaviors. It was not until I started believing in myself that my attitude changed. In order to recover from grief, you must be willing to try. In order to feel significant relief, there were several steps that I followed that truly helped put me at ease. This, for me, is important to share with you. I've been through this pain several times and there are a few lessons I learned.

STEP 1: ACKNOWLEDGE YOUR LOVED ONES AS IF THEY ARE STILL AROUND

This resolution came with much introspection. Thinking about what the research taught me, I decided that the only way to cure the immediate pain was to mimic the stimulus. So what does this mean? I came to realize that my momentary outbursts were alleviated by talking to my family members as if they were still there. Of course, I didn't do this in public settings. But when it comes to your own life, you have the power to decide how you will include them. One of the things I would do was to carry a good luck charm of my dad for comfort. Then when I was having a hard day, I would speak to him about my problems. It is difficult to explain, but this made me feel better. Each time I imagined his rational response, I would become instantly calmer.

Doing this helped me channel his good energy back into my life. This also allowed me to honor him. I found that when I was alone, living with my loved one's positivity made daily stressors become manageable. I also improved my faith in God as a born-again Christian. I had to come to the point where I was okay with not having all the answers to healing. Part of accepting this helped me do away with my "screw the world" mentality.

Of course, this seems cliché, but I promise it works. We cannot control when it is a person's time to die. We are only incapable of overcoming adversity if we lose the ability to believe in ourselves. No matter what, having some foresight and control over how we think about our loved one allows for a sense of freedom throughout the bereavement process.

STEP 2: ONE FEELING AT A TIME, ONE DAY AT A TIME

One point to consider is that feelings come in waves. They are only overwhelming if you fail to address them. The trick with doing so is making sure to process each emotion and its reaction within us, one at a time. If you try to interpret all of your negative feelings at the same time, it will probably lead to a meltdown. It is too overwhelming. Each thought left unmanaged will flood your head, making it difficult to function.

I suggest making the time to write your feelings down in a notebook or journal. As silly as that seems, it helps to provide a sense of perspective as if you are on the outside looking in. When you keep a record of this in your notebook, make a list of all your current emotions. After doing so, circle all the feelings that are irrational. For example, if your list contains these items: I am angry with myself for not saving my cousin, I feel guilty for not dying too, and it is my fault that my cousin died. The first two emotions are normal, but the last one is negative and irrational. It is justifiable to feel angry with yourself. But it is not okay to blame yourself for surviving or for making the accident happen. These are all factors that are out of your control. Everything happens for a reason and we do not have control over who lives and dies. Even if you were not in the car with your relative that night, something still may have happened. Accidents happen. In order to start the process of recovery, you must take small steps to improve the way your mind frames your beliefs surrounding the loss as well as how you cope with it.

I know this is easier said than done. But I believe that you have the power to heal. You must believe in yourself and stop trying to feel in control of all the things in the world. There is a reason why we are only in control of ourselves. We are not meant to bear the burdens of others. We can only do our best to do the right thing. And that is all that matters.

I have personally completed this exercise. For me, it became a daily catharsis. I noticed that it reduces the possibility for you to have a temper tantrum on the barista at the coffee shop, the pharmacist, waiter, or the mailman. Outsiders do not deserve to be your punching bag. If you learn how to manage your emotions as they surface, you will not explode. Nor will you become a danger to yourself or others. By following these steps, you will start to see your life back on track. And if you are not able to help yourself, do not be afraid to ask for help from a professional. It is more than okay if you do not have the strength. Others will be there at your request in your darkest hour.

STEP 3: DO NOT ISOLATE, ENGAGE

It is okay that no one comprehends why you are still grieving. And this is because it is not for anyone else but you to understand. Unfortunately, as humans we either try to discredit or shame what we don't understand rather than being open-minded and supportive. Not everyone heals according to the same timeline, so any person who believes they have the right to make these determinations, should mind their own business. Do what is best for you, no matter what the circumstances, because it is not worth sacrificing your happiness.

Part of being able to reconnect your interpersonal relationships requires knowing that no one will truly understand your emotions. So there is nothing wrong with educating them. But you want to share in a way that does not intimidate others. In plain language, this means filtering the level of morbid details you share. If they react in a way that makes you feel uncomfortable, then it's best to not discuss too much with friends that you do not know or trust.

Grief support groups help with providing comfort for those who have limited social support. Their main purpose is to gather in groups that exchange stories and commiserate through similar experiences.

The purpose of fleshing through the reactions of your friends is to recognize, as a newly grieving person, that remaining in isolation only enhances bereavement. Your friends are there to keep you busy and to prevent you ruminating all day. It is good to experience your emotions, but when you are stuck on them, you cannot make any progress. Onc of the exercises I did was writing daily letters to my loved ones. This helped me to say what I had to say without burdening the people around me.

STEP 4: KEEP TRYING

Believe it or not, this is the most important step. You cannot give up on yourself. You need to wake up each morning, treating it as a fresh start. How you deal with the loss is up to you. But just remember, the choices that you make to help yourself are what make a difference in your recovery over time. Doing nothing could be detrimental to your mental health recovery. If you incorporate at least some of these tools I mentioned, and learn more about complicated grief, the healing process becomes less intimidating.

One thing I recommend is not letting go of your self-care routines. In the midst of deep mourning, I would wear the same clothes for days, forget to brush my hair, or shower. It was difficult for me to enjoy taking care of myself without my dad around. I felt like there was no point to care. But there is! You have to continue to care for yourself, despite everything, because no one else will do that for you.

STEP 5: REMAIN POSITIVE THROUGHOUT PROGRESSIVE WITHDRAWAL

As indicated previously, the loss of a loved one mimics drug withdrawal. This makes being alone a challenge. If your symptoms of depression, panic, anxiety, nightmares, and changes in diet become too drastic, you ought to consider seeking professional help. Do not shame yourself for making the choice to reach out. It is one of the best decisions I ever made. In fact, I would not be here today if I didn't lean on therapists in a time of need.

As I was taught by my mentors, the best way to recover is to remain positive. This means working on changing your thoughts from "I don't know how I am going to get through this!" or "I just don't have it in me to get dressed and face the world without this person" and "I can't be happy because they are no longer here with me." These negative thoughts can be revised to "I know this won't be easy, but I can get through this" and "Even if I can't get dressed, I think it is better for me to face the world instead of hiding indoors." These are only some suggestions as to how to incorporate more elements of positivity into the thoughts that swarm your mind following a major loss. Adding elements of positivity will help to break up the continuity of negative thinking and the behavior associated with it.

STEP 6: BAD MEMORY SUBSTITUTION TECHNIQUE

If you are suffering from haunting thoughts of traumatic experiences that surround a loss, there is a way to combat this. Rather than focusing on those times that brought you to remember why you and your lost family member argued, focus on cancelling out those disturbing thoughts with the happy moments. These moments should be favored and should not be discounted just because there were many troubling circumstances. For instance, there are many times that my father and I argued, getting so angry at each other that we said things we didn't mean. However, after his death, I learned to put those good memories first because the bad ones just created more pain than I could reasonably handle. I was already struggling with him being gone and to add all the negativity on top of that just made it take longer to heal. You should acknowledge those memories when they come up, process them, and then think of a corresponding good time. If you create a mental inventory of all the great family vacations and happy moments, these will soon begin to replace those that are unfavorable.

STEP 7: IT IS OKAY TO BE EMOTIONAL!

When creating these steps, I have realized that it sounds counterproductive to be upset or think about the bad times with your loved one. But this is not the truth. Crying and recognizing your anger are critical to recovery. It is not productive when your worst memories are the only thing you think about. It is no one's business to tell you that you can't. It is your personal emotional journey and these steps are the stepping stones to getting better. I didn't have any help, so it has been my dream to offer what has worked for me. From the bottom of my heart, I will feel so grateful if these steps can help anyone.

References

Abnormal Grief Reactions: Complicated Mourning. (2008). *Grief Counseling and Grief Therapy.* doi:10.1891/9780826101211.0005

Bowlby, J. (1979). The Bowlby-Ainsworth attachment theory. *Behavioral and Brain Sciences, 2*(4), 637-638. doi:10.1017/s0140525x00064955

Bowlby, R. (2018). Fifty Years of Attachment Theory. *Fifty Years of Attachment Theory,* 11-26. doi:10.4324/9780429474736-2

Burkett, J. P., & Young, L. J. (2012). The behavioral, anatomical and pharmacological parallels between social attachment, love and addiction. *Psychopharmacology, 224*(1), 1 26. doi:10.1007s00213-012-2794-x

Black, D. W., & Grant, J. E. (2014). DSM-5 guidebook: The essential companion to the Diagnostic and statistical manual of mental disorders, fifth edition. American Psychiatric Publishing.

Grief Therapy: Resolving Complicated Mourning. (2008). *Grief Counseling and Grief Therapy.* doi:10.1891/9780826101211.0006

Horowitz, M. J., Siegel, B., Holen, A., Bonanno, G. A., Milbrath, C., & Stinson, C. H. (2003). Diagnostic Criteria for Complicated Grief Disorder. *Focus, 1*(3), 290-298. doi:10.1176/foc.1.3.290

Koob, G. F. (2009). Brain stress systems in the amygdala and addiction. *Brain Research, 1293,* 61-75. doi:10.1016/j.brainres.2009.03.038

Koob, G. F. (2003). Neuroadaptive mechanisms of addiction: Studies on the extended amygdala. *European Neuropsychopharmacology, 13*(6), 442-452. doi:10.1016/j.euroneuro.2003.08.005

Kubler-Ross, E. (1969). *On death and dying.* Macmillan.

Lewis, C. S., & Gang, Y. (2004). *A grief observed.* Hongsŏngsa.

Middleton, W., Raphael, B., Martinek, N., & Misso, V. (1993). Pathological grief reactions. *Handbook of Bereavement,* 44-61. doi:10.1017cbo9780511664076.004

Neimeyer, R. (2005). Grief, loss, and the quest for meaning. *Bereavement Care, 24*(2), 27-30. doi:10.1080/02682620508657628

Nestler, E. J., & Aghajanian, G. K. (1997). Molecular and Cellular Basis of Addiction. *Science, 278*(5335), 58-63. doi:10.1126/science.278.5335.58

O'Connor, M., Wellisch, D. K., Stanton, A. L., Eisenberger, N. I., Irwin, M. R., & Lieberman, M. D. (2008). Craving love? Enduring grief activates brain's reward center. *NeuroImage, 42*(2), 969-972. doi:10.1016/j.neuroimage.2008.04.256

What is Grief? (n.d.). https://hospicefoundation.org/Grief-(1)/What-to-Expect

3

THE DETERRENCE OF LOVE

> *"If we refuse to give love because we fear pain or loss, then our lives will be empty, our loss greater."*
>
> — *OPRAH WINFREY*

I was fifteen years old during the winter of 2006. I had just moved from North Jersey to South Jersey. My first culture shock took place during our abrupt move to a new town and school. Moving from suburbia to an island was more of a transition than I initially anticipated. I was hesitant, but forced to adjust from the fast life to a desolate one. This seaside town was secluded and small in comparison to what I considered home. On one side of the island was a bay and on the other was the ocean, but in between were doll-like houses for show. This change in environment did little to change my shy and naïve demeanor. Although more outgoing than before, I was still the girl learning to find her voice.

Only several weeks earlier, I had a home and family that other kids at school envied. Most of my friend's parents were already divorced, and the kids were engaging in dangerous behavior that I could not identify with, being the good girl and all. I was entirely grateful to have parents that were always loving and supportive no matter what. They never tried to buy my affection like other parents, they provided me with unconditional love. And in return, I cared for them just the same.

Then a month later, my dad began to struggle with maintaining consistent work. But this did not make me question my faith in his ability to get back on his feet. My mother was working, but it wasn't enough to pull us out of a financial hole. Being so young, I failed to comprehend that this family crisis could lead to devastating circumstances that would nearly incapacitate me mentally.

The original owner of the house had a great rapport with my parents and he adored my brother and I. He was getting older and began to demonstrate the irreversible effects of Alzheimer's Dementia. As a consequence, his daughter took over as the new landlord. She raised our rent, knowing it would be unattainable. I watched my parents fight relentlessly for us to stay there. My mother even tried to negotiate a way to buy our family time, but the owner was unyielding. She gave us an *ultimatum*: either pay the extra 1000 a month or leave within 30 days. After the 30 days, we had 3 days to move. I knew we were suffering financially for a while, but I did not understand the gravity of the situation.

I watched my parents' sense of self-worth depreciate as the clock counted down. I initially processed this pain as shock. I was not mature enough to grasp the reality of losing everything - for I had a unique physical and emotional attachment to my belongings and I was not mentally prepared to part with anything. To add to forced possession detachment, we struggled with having barely enough money for food and gas, driving around in search of a place to live. I had the fight left in me to maintain hope.

I made a choice on packing day: either allow this situation to break me or rise to the occasion. I chose to make the decisions during my parents' state of panic. I carefully and methodologically packed our most important belongings in boxes. Each garbage bag signified a piece of my past being thrown into a dark abyss. My parents made many phone calls with no progress, and with each failed attempt I saw their pride sinking deeper. Social services were useless, as always. I watched them help people who did not need it. Because of that, I resented all of their staff and the families before us in a line that failed to prevent our family of 4 from being homeless.

Despite these challenges, I motivated my father to not give up. Even now, I hope he appreciates the inner strength I acquired during those moments. For I, too, saw a part of him I'd never seen before - the part of him that becomes vulnerable when faced with hardship. The man, with impenetrable courage, was capable of showing pain. Even though I know he fought his emotions as hard as his clenched fists and jaw would allow, his red eyes gave it all away. He sobbed on the inside. I could tell by the way he silently held his head down under his hat.

By day three, a miracle occurred. I finished packing the house. We stood outside reflecting on our next step while our boxes waited patiently inside the warm house. We were frozen stiffer than ice that winter by the silence of crucial decision-making.

Before relocating, we were forced to leave behind five cats and most of our belongings. Even my favorite clothes, toys, and books had to be discarded. We were only able to bring the items that fit in our car. I failed to understand how much being petless would impact me. I cherished my beautiful cats, Angel, Sandy, and her 3 kittens. They were always there to greet and comfort me after not only rough days at school but also the best ones. The thought of not having them on either of those occasions gave me intense distress. Thank God my mom was able to place all of them since they were all already fixed and had all their shots.

Looking back, I realized those belongings were pieces of my identity.

It was earth shattering, leaving behind almost everything, especially when the shock made the sharp transition into harsh reality. My dad worked hard to show me I was worthy of reward, and when I studied, I earned his attention and respect. He taught me how to work for what I wanted, and that is why I fell in love with this place. I was a part of it and it was a part of me. I felt like my heart had been ripped through my chest and stepped on. There was little I could do to rectify the situation. So I did the only thing I could, which was to keep moving forward, no matter how hard I'd fallen. I knew I would recover only if I picked my head up and did my best with the new adjustments ahead.

From my first real encounter with heartbreak, I learned that nothing you love lasts forever, especially if it's something you cherish. I spent years building a bond with this place, only to have it shattered by external circumstances.

As we drove away to look for somewhere else to live, I realized that a piece of my heart stayed behind with our abandoned property.

While still in school everyday mom and dad spent their

time looking for a place to call home. We ended up staying at a hotel for 30 days. Somehow, we were able to survive. On the weekends I would go with my parents, driving to check out the list of potential houses and rentals. Eventually we visited this quiet apartment located between the bay and the ocean on the barrier island. As luck would have it, the realtor happened to be standing outside as we passed by. He let us take a look at the 3 bedroom. With no amenities, it was far below what we were accustomed to. It had to do, given there were no financial options. This seaside home was uncomfortably quiet, especially in the middle of the winter. I knew that my connection with this place would be like seeds that require water to promote their growth.

Following a few weeks of hesitation, I became accustomed to the new surroundings and tried to adapt to a new group of friends. Little did I know that I was going to find myself falling in love for the very first time. And I certainly was not emotionally prepared for the other firsts that were about to take place.

My first week at the new school, Central Regional High, I met this charming young man. He had a great personality and was a football player. So of course, he had an attractive muscular physique complimented by a gorgeous smile. One day, he saw me walking down the hallway and he came over to say hello. It was easy enough to notice me, being the new girl and all. One small introduction later, he asked me out on a date. It didn't take much convincing for me to accept his offer. To be honest, I failed to remember my exact response, being so nervous about looking stupid in front of the popular guy in school.

With much excitement and anticipation, our first date was all that I had dreamed of at fifteen years old. If I recall correctly, I intentionally neglected to inform my parents of this date. I knew they were overly protective. Besides, even if I asked nicely, they would have said "absolutely not." He took me to the towns' best attraction - the Seaside Heights boardwalk overlooking the beach. When we stopped walking, I noticed we were on the pier just across from the Ferris wheel. I was so excited that he went out of his way to make me feel special. I was in awe that there was almost no one around, except the person to operate the ride. He was the first and only person who offered to show me around town. On the big wheel in the sky, I felt like I was high off life, smiling so hard it actually hurt. When we stepped off the ride, we skipped around the arcade for a while taking pictures of ourselves in the photo booth. In the back of my mind, I felt guilty sneaking off without the permission of my parents. But I couldn't help but feel the thrill of doing something I wasn't supposed to do. He got my spirits lifted so much that he made me giggle whenever he started talking. I even had butterflies when he looked me in the eyes.

As that first night together came to an end, he pulled me towards him and kissed me for the first time. My body was covered in pins and needles. Just the touch of his hand made my heart race out of my chest. With the first touch of his lips, my body was overcome by shivers. He had the most sensual way of moving from the top lip to the bottom one. I felt a tingling sensation from head to toe as he continued touching the side of my face. He had the power to take me to the moon and back in just a few seconds. I felt like I had been blessed with the most amazing man. I was certain I was falling in love.

On our next few dates, I was so giddy with excitement because I was unable to believe that my first date was every little girl's dream turned into reality. He constantly made me giggle like a kid on Christmas morning opening up their first present. I was elated that a man was interested in me enough to ask me to be his girlfriend.

After several months, I began to question how well I knew this man. I was unaware of his past or his real personality outside of our relationship. I was so infatuated that I invested all my trust without hesitation. I believed every word out of his mouth was genuine. I was confident his intentions were good. In my mind, all of his love letters signified commitment, trust, and honesty.

The problem was that I was incapable of identifying his true intentions because I was blinded by love. In retrospect, I should have questioned his need to rush into saying "I love you." In my innocent nature, and certainly against my parents' advice, I gave my virginity to this man.

It wasn't long before I began to realize that every word out of my boyfriend's mouth was a twisted version of the truth. He wanted me to only see this false image that he created for himself. After speaking to his friends about his whirlwind romance, I began to learn the painful truth. Almost every word he told me was verified as lies. Yet my foolish heart and unrelenting ability to forgive set me up for heartbreak. I saw the good in this man in spite of the mounting evidence against him. I used his honorable qualities to dismiss the months of manipulation. I repeatedly took him back over the coming months, hurting myself more each time.

Eventually, it came to the point where the deception became embedded so far underneath the truth that I no longer recognized the man I thought I loved. My family was there to support me amidst the emotional pain and disappointment, leading them to intervene. Because of their support and my own strength, I was able to let him go. Since that was my first experience with what I thought was love, I was heartbroken. I was angry with myself for falling for a facade. From that moment forward, I developed an internal distrust towards men. I realized that any man would be capable of saying what I wanted to hear. Believing those words would allow them to take what they wanted from me.

The distrust and fear were deepened by my later reunion with him. Late one winter night, I snuck out of the house with my best friend. When we got to his apartment, they were immediately participating in drinking games. I cheered this on, since I was not experienced with alcohol. As it turns out, she had way too much hard liquor. It was not long before she started to turn green and vomit all over the floor. Trying to be a gentleman, he escorted her to his bathroom fully clothed. When I went to check on her moments later, she was fully nude and he was touching her inappropriately.

From our previous discussions, my best friend had a bad habit of disrobing under the influence of alcohol. The problem was that she made a choice to drink in excess. To make matters worse, he decided to take advantage of her while she was too mentally incapacitated to understand the consequences of her actions.

It was this experience that forced me to realize how much I haphazardly trusted potential love interests. It took me a long time to allow any male close enough to hurt me.

A secondary consequence of this first so-called love, was that our most intimate exchanges were shared with his circle of friends. His friends did not have good intentions either. One man in particular truly impacted my life in a negative way. As much as it pains me to reveal the details, it's important for me to do so in order to break the chains that shackle me.

This troubled man befriended my brother along with the man I was dating. One night he came over to visit my brother to play video games on the Xbox. I was dead asleep in the room next door. Earlier in the day, I had participated in a track meet. That particular track meet, I ran in 3 events and the 4th event was a pole-vault meet. During the race, I struggled to fight through a lingering hip and knee injury. This limited my mobility on and off the field. Despite the immense pain I suffered, I remained in the registered relays out of my commitment to my coach and the team.

It took every ounce of energy for me to eat that night, since subtle movements seemed to agitate my pain. Shortly after dinner, I turned the light off and passed out. I was finally in a deep sleep where none of the suffering I endured that day could reach me. Before I could understand what was going on, I was awakened to this man on top of me. He must have broken into my room without me noticing. I was so frightened at that moment, my body froze. I was able to beg him to please stop despite choking on my tears. I begged him to leave several more times, but my arms were pinned to my sides by the way he had all of this body weight pressed against me. All I could see in front of me was the dark green glare in his eyes seeking to get what he wanted from me. In between forceful kisses, I gasped for air. And with each breath, I held back the urge to gag from his yellow and brown decaying teeth that wreaked of cigarettes. Even more putrid was the stench of his greasy hair brushing against my face as he kept forcefully touching me down there. And that's the place no one's allowed to go without permission.

Even though my family was asleep in the rest of the house, they were not awakened by my cries. Every utterance I made, I pushed as hard as I could to draw attention. But there was this vocal paralysis prompted by my fear. Every effort my mouth attempted to make was met with a deafening silence. I felt as though I was yelling, but no actual noise came out.

After the kisses, he began touching my breasts. His efforts to touch the rest of my body felt like sharp splinters meeting my skin at each intersection. He pleaded for me to let him penetrate me as he unzipped his pants, exposing himself. He was already so aroused by the thought of my resistance. This was compounded by the fact that I was only 16 years old and he was over the age of 18.

As he laid bare above me with my arms still restrained by his top half, he quickly pulled down my red spandex shorts. It was then I fought even harder to gain control over my hands. As he positioned himself, I was able to make a negotiation with him. I realized that if I touched him with only my hands, he would not go inside me.

With each stroke of my hand against him, I felt utterly and truly powerless. Tears endlessly flowed down my face, and I continued to choke on my own phlegm. A giant piece of my innocence had been stolen because I made a choice to comply rather than fight harder for my life. With each tug back and forth towards him, I lost every ounce of optimism that the old me would return again. In order to protect myself, I went into another place mentally. When he was finished, the only thing that remained of me was an empty vessel. The part of me that evacuated would never return again.

I remember little after the assault; except he took my towel to clean himself. He left me there with no regard for what he'd done. Although I don't remember when he left, I was so relieved that he was gone. This was over for him. But it wasn't over for me. I was still motionless, unable to process, and unable to think. My brother came in to check on me. As I tried to utter the words "he hurt me, help," but nothing was audible to my brother. Because he didn't understand my mumbles, he left, returning to his own room.

I knew that if I woke my mom and dad, we wouldn't have a sexual assault investigation, but a murder scene. So, I went back to sleep and awoke the next morning so afraid to say a word about the previous night. I felt like no one would believe me because I had innocently flirted with him the day before. He had even seen me in my tight spandex track uniform. I felt like I was to blame in every possible way. Make matters worse, I didn't yell loud enough for someone to hear me. I believed it was all my fault because I made that negotiation with him. I knew that would be construed as consent.

It took me until the next day to break the news to my mother. I was filled with shame and my spirit was so broken, recounting this event required immense courage. My mother broke the news to my father, and it truly devastated him. He was angry that I didn't wake him up and say something. He was also gravely upset that he didn't have the opportunity to make this better.

Later that evening, my mother called the police. The crime scene investigation unit came to the house to process my entire room and document the scene. Everyone in my family was brought down to the police station that night, and we gave our statements. The next day they took my attacker into custody. According to his account of the event, the encounter was entirely consensual. I didn't scream loud enough for my own brother to verify that I actually was assaulted against my will. It bothered me so much that my brother did not even acknowledge that I was hurt by this man. Instead, he said he did hear a noise, but was not sure if it was consistent with a sexual assault. He was playing his Xbox and was unsure about how to interpret the sounds coming from my room. I know he was trying to be honest. But because of this, the police department decided to drop the charges against this man. In addition, my ex-boyfriend was joining the police force, so this only worked against me. This was particularly devastating for me, given that the towel he cleaned himself with verified my story. And if he was on top of me when I was sleeping, how could I possibly consent to something that was already happening before I could stop it. I even went to a lawyer to see if we could get the charges brought back against him, but he said there was no changing the decision of the police department. I was hurt that he did not fight for me, and that's what he was paid to do.

It was this experience that made me feel as if my words truly had no value or power at all. Even if I was able to scream would that really change the outcome? I still believed that I would not be taken seriously because my attacker was experienced with assaulting younger girls and getting away with it. Unfortunately, he was well versed in the discourse used for evading the law. Four months earlier, I had witnessed two separate assaults on girls younger than me. Had I known that I would be the next target, I would have avoided this man at all costs and certainly would not have allowed him in our home.

I truly know that if this assault were to happen today, there would be a different result. I would have been rewarded with justice thanks to the new found support of the #metoo movement. So, I share this lesson as a learning experience. As women, we have come such a long way, and I hope that my story provides additional support for the progress we still need to make.

IMMEDIATE EMOTIONAL PROCESSING

At the time, I was a fit track and field athlete and pole vaulter. To put it modestly, I was in great physical condition and flaunted my attributes by wearing crop tops, tight jeans and shorts. I was proud to show off the body I invested the time to earn. Being so young, I believed it was my fault for dressing in a way that demanded negative attention. I convinced myself that my mature wardrobe choices made me vulnerable. Immediately after the assault, I shamed myself for dressing provocatively. I thought maybe it wouldn't have happened if I made it a priority to dress appropriately around men.

Naturally, because I failed to understand these concepts, I was prone to being taken advantage of. The problem with my thinking at the time was that I did not understand that I could respect myself and dress any way that I liked. Being myself is not an invite to be attacked in a sexual manner. It is true that men take a harmless smile from a pretty girl and equate that to sex, but that is not a reflection on the woman. I now can understand, it was not my fault that he decided to come after me that night.

Feeling so powerless before and after the attack, I felt like my voice would never be worthy of listening to. Even if I was able to express my emotions, I believed it would not change the outcome. My sentiments concerning this matter extended to all situations, not just those where I felt threatened. It took time for me to allow anyone to overpower me. And when I was in a dangerous situation, I used my anger from this situation to defend myself. During later sexual encounters, I felt it was necessary to maintain control over my partner. If I did not have power over my significant other, there was no balance in the relationship.

Regardless of my actions, this young man had a history of assaulting under age females. So there was a high probability of me being taken advantage of, even if I had been dressed appropriately. In my opinion, that man came to my house with the intention of befriending my brother so that he could have his way with me. As easy as it was to blame myself, I cannot take full responsibility. This act was premeditated irrespective of the influence of my prior behavior. I could not continue to guilt myself for actions that can't be changed.

My first boyfriend allowed me to learn that actions validate words. That is how we evaluate accountability and honesty. This is important for getting to know someone. Love and trust work together with the ability to verify that each action can be accounted for. In other words, promises should be followed through prior to investing more time and emotion. It is important to get to know someone before calling them your boyfriend or even using the words "I love you". Even though I learned from my first mistake, I still was inclined to give men chances that did not deserve it.

When it comes to the sexual assault, I now see it happened for a reason. I was meant to learn how to protect myself not just in a physical sense, but to be aware of their male intentions prior to exposing my vulnerable side. He reminded me to fight through my fear of speaking up in a terrifying situation.

I also sought to show other girls in my dormitory how to trust their instincts when going out to parties. Even though the police didn't help me or use the DNA evidence to make a conviction, what mattered most was that I survived that painful experience. The police denying me help caused me to fight even harder to become an advocate for women's rights. Although he stole a piece of my innocence, he also inspired me to become the best version of myself.

STEPS TOWARDS SEXUAL ASSAULT RECOVERY

STOP BLAMING YOURSELF

No matter how intense your feelings of self-blame and guilt may be, you have to remind yourself that you are the victim of the situation. But being the victim does not equate to permanent powerlessness. You are now a survivor! You have been given the gift of adversity for the purpose of self-expansion. You can be who you are without feeling ashamed of the past. The minute you stop blaming yourself for our situation, you can gain a newfound sense of power over our future.

DON'T BE AFRAID TO SPEAK OUT

Although it may be difficult to talk about what happened to you, it is important to speak out and report your story to the authorities. That gives you the ability to seek justice. Even if you are embarrassed, it is best to share as much detail as possible so that the police can catch your attacker. More importantly, you must continue to fight for yourself no matter how threatened or intimidated you feel.

FORGIVE YOURSELF!

Many survivors of sexual assault believe that they are to blame for what happened to them. That cannot be further from the truth. Just because you dressed a certain way or smiled too brightly, that does not justify someone hurting you. No means no and that can change at any moment in time. If you initially agreed to be intimate with someone, but they suddenly make you uncomfortable, your consent can change. If you express no permission for sexual penetration, you are not to blame. The person trying to move forwards against your wishes is automatically in the wrong, for that is a direct violation of your personal space.

Because of the #metoo movement, there is a larger platform to share your story without the victim blaming.

MAKE CLEAR CONSENT

This situation taught me to never allow for ambiguity when it comes to physical interaction with men. I now make sure to discuss what my feelings are regarding sex and my body. If those things are not respected in the slightest sense, I do not allow further contact. I encourage other women to do the same. Unfortunately, men are not good with ambiguity. If we do not say “NO” in the most obvious way, it becomes open for interpretation. Furthermore, I am here to remind you that you can revoke consent at any time. If you no longer feel comfortable engaging on the physical level, you have the right to stop it at any time. If this is not respected, it is subject to punishment in the eyes of the law.

REBUILD YOUR IDENTITY

It is easy to feel like your attacker took a part of you, making you afraid to express yourself or be happy again. But I am here to tell you to not give them that power. For many years, I felt like no one would care because the police did nothing for me. The police favored the lies of my attacker. If you share the same story, it is important that you continue to live in a way that defines the strength in your spirit. By this I mean don't be afraid to live your life, have friends, and follow your dreams because of what happened.

But what does this rebuilding actually entail? I mean start each day like you're laying bricks to put your own house back together. From the first day, do what makes you happy, as difficult as that may be. One of the things I did was find ways to express myself through my writing or singing. I would find a way to share that with someone close to me and that would inspire me to continue on this journey of self-reparation. Then from the second day onward, you can give yourself power by putting your needs on top of the to-do list. I would try to hide in my job or school work, but that prevented me from acknowledging my emotional needs. The more I forced myself to do what was best for me, the more I grew. Keep focusing on doing what makes you feel like a human again, not the one that was ravaged by an animal. And eventually, you will start to see a new image of yourself emerge through what you thought could no longer be identified.

POSITIVE AFFIRMATIONS

During this arduous recovery, I recommend learning how to incorporate positive affirmations into your life. This means replacing the negative, self-deprecating thoughts with something good. For example, rather than saying "I am never going to be respected by men and I am unworthy of love" you should say, "I am worthy of love and respect."

Other examples consist of statements such as this: "I am smart, I am good enough, and I am beautiful on the inside and out."

Replacing your bouts of negativity with these alternatives will help you to have faith, courage, and confidence in yourself again. In fact, I can guarantee that what you had been saying to yourself before was overly critical and untrue.

REFRAMING MY PERSPECTIVE

Reflection of those experiences leads me to understand their significance. From the first time I was homeless, I learned the value of appreciating what I have. I realized after losing so many material belongings that they are just that. Those possessions, even with sentimental value, are tied to a memory. Even if I lose the object of my affection, the connection to that memory remains. Losing our home and my innocence led to a new beginning, and a chance to learn about the fundamentals about life. By cognitively reframing the situation, I see that I've gained an inner strength and motivation to thrive.

There is a sense of peace that follows heartache, assault,

and homelessness. You just have to take the time to change the way you perceive.

References

Lives Quotes (85 Quotes). (n.d.).
https://quotescover.com/topics/lives/page/4

4

THE TORTURE OF ABANDONMENT

> *"He wanted to leave the past a few hundred miles down the road, shake it off like dust. But that was the problem with the past. It kept finding him."*
>
> — *SUZANNE WOODS FISHER, THE KEEPER: A NOVEL*

Without a doubt, I was a daddy's girl. Overall, I had a valuable relationship with my parents. But my dad was always physically present as my teacher, inspiration, support system, protector, and cheerleader. Little did I know, he was at war with many inner demons. When I was a child, I wanted to be the tough girl he could never give up on. And I was, but there were signs as early as three to six years old that something was amiss. When I would come home from preschool, I noticed he would sit by the TV, always physically present, but mentally disengaged. Frequently accompanying his hand on the arm rest of the couch was a can covered in a blue sleeve. I could smell the alcohol seeping through his pores. Over time, I began to make the connection that he was playing with me less and prioritizing sitting on the couch watching his TV shows.

For the most part, I did not take offense at this. Even as a child I knew it was nearly impossible to have the one hundred percent, undivided attention of an adult. I wasn't selfish. Actually, I was quite independent, being able to entertain myself with books and dolls. But there was one incident where I began to notice that my attachment to him was not as secure as I originally believed.

My brother and I were wrestling around on the top of the two bunk beds in our room. Somehow, I ended up falling off, landing directly on the back of my head. This crash into the floor literally knocked my lights out. I couldn't see straight for ten minutes at least, but somehow, I managed to stumble my way downstairs. My dad was in his usual spot on the couch. I was sobbing, holding my head. I told him I fell, and right after those words came out, vomit came rushing out of my mouth and onto the ground. He didn't seem to believe me, and I didn't understand why. If he did, he would have jumped up out of his seat to do something to help. Instead, he cracked open another can, sighed heavily, took the old one, crushed it, and replaced the sleeve with the new one. Then, he grabbed some ice from the refrigerator and told me to put it on my head.

I knew something was wrong. I felt like a bother to him at that moment. I thought to myself, mom would have reacted much differently. Maybe he was afraid to look like the irresponsible adult. I could read his facial expressions, and they told me he wasn't happy with himself. That drink in his hand seemed to make decisions for him in these moments. The can always seemed to be glued to his hand when sitting in that spot, causing my needs to become secondary. I could see the internal battle taking place within his soul. He wanted to take accountability, but even he was hesitant to interact his fears directly. He was afraid of facing the reasons that made him drink. I realized that beer became a security blanket preventing him from facing reality.

In between periods of hard work to maintain sobriety over the years, he succumbed to his alcohol addiction. With each relapse came changes in behavior. I would notice coming home from school and he would not come out of his truck. In the beginning, he would come home and stay inside. I think he was embarrassed to be drinking heavily inside the house. Plus, my mom would not have tolerated that level of misbehavior with her two kids. Because of this, he resorted to drinking beer outdoors.

Then the unthinkable started to happen. He would stay out, disappear, and no one could find him. Mom and I made it our mission to keep searching, no matter what. My mom followed him a few times and realized that he was going to bad neighborhoods and park the truck on side streets so that he couldn't be found for hours. On one occasion, he checked into a motel and my mother had the truck towed.

Devastated wasn't the word. He didn't show that night. He took a cab back to our house the next morning and the walk of shame to the front door. It was clear he was hungover in more ways than one. And I had to explain to my brother what happened. This was the first time my brother and I were exposed to this kind of behavior. We all expected the best from dad.

Later that night after dad slept off some of the hangover, my brother and I heard the arguments heating up between our parents. She insisted that he answer the questions about whether or not he was cheating. Initially, mom was in denial and thought whatever he was doing was just to get drugs. In response to his actions that day, my brother and I grabbed onto each other and cried for a long time. This is the first time we realized that our dad was not the man we thought he was. Regardless of his mistakes, we loved him so much. I believe that's why this moment changed our expectations and made us disappointed.

Being hurt did not change the fact that I wanted the

best for my father. I knew he was more than capable as an honorably discharged Marine from the Vietnam Era, and the only man that could fight anything. From his drunken episodes, monologues of his past began to emerge. It was in those moments, I saw the unfiltered version of dad, not the one who hides behind the beer can and the bill of his hat. Most of his grievances stemmed from his difficult childhood. He saw his brother, John, early on engaging in drug use - and he was the good kid, athlete and star student. This served as a major source of pain and disappointment for him.

In addition, his parents did not express love physically or verbally. They both struggled with an addiction of some sort. I'm sure this caused him to feel unworthy of love, recognition, and especially undeserving of praise. He was younger than me when he told his father that he found out his mother was cheating, but he seemed unperturbed since he also was involved in extramarital affairs. As a teenager, this affected his perception of trust, honesty, love, identity, and existence.

No matter who you are, having stable parents keeps you grounded. So as can be imagined, this ripped the carpet from under him, creating a sense of instability. He tried so hard to be good, but with no one to reward him for making the right choices, he began to experiment with drugs and alcohol use.

Around his late 30s, his mother died tragically as a

result of a massive brain tumor. This had an enormous impact on his outlook on life, and it affected his brother as well. His brother died at an early age of a drug overdose. I'm sure the impact of both deaths was traumatizing. Looking back at my time with him, I'm guessing the hurt he endured led to self-medicating.

I suspect that his childhood traumas caused him to feel abandoned emotionally. So when he began to struggle with his own addiction, he inevitably ended up doing the same to me.

From this experience, I feared being abandoned again. I was afraid to love someone so much because that came with the risk of loss. The expectation of grief and emotional void has made my dating life quite turbulent. I had built a brick wall surrounding my heart to prevent myself from committing. It seemed easier to control when and how I lost, rather than remain exposed and vulnerable to manipulation.

Because of my father's decades-long battles, he began to develop dementia. This was due to liver failure, causing the unfiltered body toxins to reach his brain. As this began to happen, it only exacerbated the years of emotional abandonment I endured.

DIGESTING DEMENTIA

Months after my father's passing, I was on this journey to understand what led to my father's demise. I thought that sharing this knowledge would be helpful to others in that same situation. And perhaps understanding his illness would lead me to a path of spiritual enlightenment, and a release of residual resentments related to needing a father. It was critical for me to obtain a sense of the nature of his disease. While I had familiarity with forms of degenerative dementia in college, learning about it and living it are two separate concepts.

One of the reasons my dad suffered such memory loss so rapidly is because of a prior traumatic brain injury. In the 1980s, my dad had a major accident at work. He fell 45 ft. off a roof and lost around 66% of his cognitive functioning. When this is combined with a history of smaller concussions, and a 30-year history of drug and alcohol abuse, as well as periods of being sober, his brain and body began to disintegrate quickly. Given my personal investigation into these matters, there is so much I would be honored to share with those experiencing a similar situation with a loved one.

WHAT IS ALCOHOL-RELATED DEMENTIA?

Alcohol-related dementia (ARD) is a disease that exists in many forms. Sadly, ARD may be considered a silent epidemic because this condition does not discriminate. ARD can target anyone with a history of chronic alcohol consumption concurrent with other factors such as prior head trauma, age, and sex. Susceptibility may increase proportionally to changes in frequency, duration, and dose of alcohol consumption over time (Gupta & Warner, 2008). In fact, Harper (1998) reported that chronic alcoholics demonstrate significant loss of brain tissue compared to controls. Overall white brain matter is affected, with reduction of the number of cortical neurons in the superior frontal cortex, hypothalamus and cerebellum. ARD has widespread effects targeting many brain regions, which becomes further complicated by other comorbidities.

ALCOHOL RELATED TOXICITY

1. NEUROTOXICITY

Long-term alcohol use increases toxins such as ammonia and manganese, which contribute to encephalopathy, or brain swelling (Gupta & Warner, 2008). Because of liver cirrhosis, toxins that would be metabolized normally cannot be degraded. Dahlberg and Colleagues (2011) provided a more detailed account of how these toxins reach the brain. Their research demonstrated that these ammonia toxins traveled through the cerebrospinal fluid (CSF) causing brain swelling and cortical matter shrinkage. These ammonia toxins in return form abscesses surrounded by capsules that contain reactive astrocytes (structural support for brain cells) and fibrous tissue. However, these capsules did not serve as a diffusion barrier and distributed to cortical, cerebellar, parietal, and occipital regions altering neurotransmission and astrocytic potassium handling. Patients suffered from disorientation, expressive aphasia (disorder of communication), seizures, or fevers depending on the brain region affected. In addition to liver failure, Dahlberg postulated that abscesses become problematic when toxins breach the capsule and penetrate cell membranes.

2. EXCITOTOXICITY

Another outcome of chronic alcohol intake is inhibition of N-methyl-D-aspartate (NMDA) and up-regulation of the NMDA receptor subtype, resulting in glutamatergic excitotoxicity and high levels of intracellular calcium (Ridley et al., 2013). The neurotransmitter glutamate, responsible for regulating excitation, becomes toxic in high amounts. Support for this neurotoxicity hypothesis emerged from animal studies, which demonstrated that dose related ethanol-induced damage to the hippocampus, hypothalamus, and cerebellum corresponded with impairments in memory and learning (Brust et al., 2010; Crews et al., 2004).

NEUROPSYCHOLOGICAL COMPARISONS BETWEEN FORMS OF DEMENTIA

Obtaining an ARD diagnosis may lead to some setbacks. The primary concern is distinguishing alcohol induced pathology from brain damage due to the alcoholic lifestyle (i.e., vitamin deficiency, malnutrition, head trauma, liver disease, diabetes) (Vetreno et al., 2011). ARD becomes progressive when alcohol use persists, exacerbating memory loss, neurotoxicity, and hepatic encephalopathy (Harper, 1998). Because these deficits are widespread, ARD can be difficult to identify.

Calderon and colleagues (2001) characterized the most common forms of dementia. Alzheimer's Dementia (AD) may be diagnosed by overall deficits in attentional function, memory, and difficulty with visuospatial tasks. As the disease progresses, patients become incontinent, are often found wandering, and experience difficulty accessing long-term memories. Dementia with the presence of Lewy Bodies (DLB) and Beta-Amyloid 42 plaques may cause tissue necrosis (death) within the cerebral cortex, brainstem nuclei, substantia nigra (SN), locus coeruleus (LC), and components of the basal forebrain cholinergic system (BFCS). These cholinergic systems are important because they play a role in learning and memory.

The clinical features of DLB include a cortical dementia with fluctuating confusion, spontaneous parkinsonism, and great difficulty with visuospatial and visuoperceptual ability. By this time, cognitive and memory impairments may be irreparable. Compared to AD, patients with ARD perform better on semantic tasks and on verbal memory recognition tasks. However, some patients with ARD are unlikely to demonstrate symptoms of language impairment (Oslin et al.,1997).

HEPATIC ENCEPHALOPATHY

Hepatic Encephalopathy (HE) is a form of ARD recognized by the progression of liver cirrhosis. High levels of serum ammonia become mediated by reduced hepatic clearance, which correlates with the severity of acute HE (Butterworth, 1993; 1987). Other toxins derived from the gut contribute to this disease process (Butterworth, 2003;1994; Van Theil et al.,1985; Zaki et al., 1983). As summarized in the above section, persistence of liver failure leads to the development of hyperammonia and neurotoxic injury to the brain, which results in brain swelling. As a consequence of these metabolic changes, RNA degradation may occur (Butterworth, 1987; Hazell & Butterworth, 1999; Sheedy et al., 2012).

WERNICKE'S ENCEPHALOPATHY & KORSAKOFF'S SYNDROME

Wernicke's encephalopathy (WE) occurs as a result of Thiamine B1 deficiency. This is due to inadequate nutritional intake in addition to the inhibitory effects on thiamine absorption through the gastrointestinal tract and T1 activation via phosphorylation. The symptoms of this kind of deficiency are associated with altered mental status, ataxia, and ophthalmoplegia (Todd et al., 1999). WE can be caused by nutritional deficiency alone, in the absence of dependence and abuse. In the presence of alcohol however, thiamine transport is compromised across the blood-brain barrier, and damages apoenzymes (a protein that forms an active enzyme by combination with a coenzyme), increasing the T1 levels needed for metabolism (Thomson et al., 2012). WE has an acute onset with the presence of ocular abnormalities, gait incoordination, and motor problems (Sechi & Serra, 2007). As WE worsens, it is possible to develop Korsakoff's syndrome (KS). KS is a disorder that is principally characterized by severe memory defects, in particular a striking loss of working memory that accompanies relatively little loss of reference memory (Victor et al., 1971; Sechi & Serra, 2007). Patients with KS are likely to demonstrate symptoms of anterograde amnesia and are unable to recall recent occurrences, despite retaining information that is implicit. As a result of this, KS patients are able to acquire motor skills and develop conditioned responses to environmental stimuli (Fama et al., 2006).

For those who experience an ongoing battle with alcohol use, it may be difficult to quit. Acute withdrawal in long-term alcoholics results in tremors, hallucinations, seizures, agitation, and fluctuating levels of alertness (Ridley et al., 2013). Over 75% of autopsied chronic alcoholics have significant brain damage and over 50% of detoxified alcoholics display some degree of learning and memory impairment (Vetreno et al., 2011). If ARD exists prior to withdrawal, it is probable that these symptoms will persist after maintaining sobriety. Although current research provides little inspiration for patient recovery, there are ways to combat the causes of ARD.

With all disorders that affect the brain, there is a spectrum of severity. If impairments are moderate, there still may be a chance for improvement. In order to help patients with ARD, we must first face the stigma against alcoholics head-on. More often than not, doctors and clinicians assume that the choice to drink alcohol should be punished by lack of support and proper treatment. Whether the person diagnosed with ARD decides to get clean, we as a society should stand behind them one hundred percent. We are all part of the problem. By calling someone a "drunk" we are making them feel unworthy of help, compassion, and empathy. If we can take a moment to understand life through the eyes of an alcoholic, perhaps we can acquire the ability to be sympathetic. Whether or not a chronic alcoholic requests treatment, they do need it. It is our duty as a society to provide that assistance with no judgment and the utmost support.

Steps towards recovery:

- Stop drinking. Attend a rehab facility that is geared towards the needs of the patient by using an individualized treatment plan. Depending on prior mental health history, the patient may require intense psychotherapy with psychotropic medicines as an adjunct to counseling. It is important that addiction and mental health issues are being adequately managed.
- Consult a general medical physician for evaluation of overall health status. If there are pre-existing conditions, it would be useful to obtain a referral for a specialist, (i.e., cardiologist if a heart condition surfaces). If ARD is still moderate, consult another physician experienced with alcohol related conditions.
- Visit a Neurologist for an accurate assessment

and diagnosis regarding memory loss. A Neuropsychologist can further evaluate cognitive impairment and formulate specific treatment plans to improve deficits.

- As a family member, it is critical to remain SUPPORTIVE and compassionate with unconditional love. Most importantly, be by their side every step of the way no matter what obstacles you may endure as a family. This is how genuine recovery begins and is maintained. Do not allow your feelings of anger and bitterness to interfere with the recovery process. If there are issues that need to be addressed, it is best to do that within family counseling where you have a proper platform to work through your issues without causing more damage and resentment.

Towards the last three months of his life, I learned to understand where he was coming from. He talked to me from a place of clarity and sobriety. He explained that his past had been traumatic, and his parents surrounded him with addiction and alcoholism. Those factors contributed to his condition. He kept trying to break free, but relapsed time and time again because of the behavioral patterns he witnessed as a child. If doing drugs, cheating, and manipulation are the tools you are given, those are what you use to survive. Most importantly, I began to realize that my dad was struggling with a disease. I now know he did not choose to abandon me. It was a consequence of his illness. Because of this, I am learning to forgive what happened between us in the past.

Furthermore, I realized that it is important for me to figure out how to heal so I don't wind up being an emotionally unavailable parent. Therefore, the following section is dedicated to the work I put into defeat my feelings of abandonment.

DEFEATING ABANDONMENT

Learn about the history of the one who abandoned you: Finding out about my father's history in terms of family, mental health, and traumatic experiences enabled me understand what factors led to his emotional void. Because of his background, I have been able to learn that he really did not have the proper upbringing to be successful in a family dynamic. Despite this, I know that he tried to do the best he could to physically be there for me as much as possible. With this newfound knowledge, I am able to release my anger towards him.

Stop blaming yourself: When you are struggling with these feelings, it is important to realize that it is not your fault. You do not have the power to change how a person responds or connects to you. Most likely, the person responsible for your pain is not in control of their subconscious motivations for abandoning others.

Break the Cycle: The worst thing that you can do is hurt someone else the same way you were. As hard as it is, you must fight the urge to disappear from a partner or friend's life. Forcing yourself to stick it out provides them with the opportunity to build a sense of trust. If you do not give others a chance, you may be missing out on genuine connections.

Remain Open and Vulnerable: It is so easy to run or shut down, but this is not practical. The more you put up a brick wall of protection, the longer you will feel lonely and unloved. To change this, you must take the time to be honest and truthful about what happened to you. Revealing your past troubles will help a potential mate or friend understand what they need to do to help you recover.

Leave Your Past Where It Belongs: Sometimes we tend to allow what happened in the past to dictate our future relationships with others. But the reality is that everyone is different. You can't punish someone for the mistakes made by others in the past. When you meet someone new, it is okay to start fresh. Remove all your preconceived notions about the men in your life that hurt you because there are good people out there with the right intentions.

References

Brust JC: Ethanol and cognition: indirect effects, neurotoxicity, and neuroprotection: a review. *Int J Environ Res Public Health*, 2010; 7:1540-1557.

Butterworth RF. Cerebral dysfunction in chronic alcoholism: role of alcoholic liver disease. *Alcohol Suppl.* 1994; 2:259–265

Butterworth RF, Giguere JF, Michaud J, Lavoie J, Layrargues GP. Ammonia: key factor in the pathogenesis of hepatic encephalopathy. *Neurochem Pathol.* 1987; 6(1–2):1–12.

Butterworth RF. Portal-systemic encephalopathy: a disorder of neuron-astrocytic metabolic trafficking. *Dev Neurosci.* 1993; 15(3–5):313–319.

Crews FT, Collins MA, Dlugos C, Littleton J, Wilksons L, Neafsey EJ, Pentney R, Snell LD, Tabakoff B, Zou J, Noronha A: Alcohol-induced neurodegeneration: when, where and why? *Alcohol Clin Exp Res,* 2004; 28:350-364.

Dahlberg D, Ivanovic J, Hassel B. Toxic levels of ammonia in human brain abscess. *J Neurosurg,* 2016; 124: 854-860.

Fama, R., Pfefferbaum, A., & Sullivan, E. V. (2006). Visuoperceptual Learning in Alcoholic Korsakoff Syndrome. *Alcoholism: Clinical and Experimental Research, 30*(4), 680-687. doi:10.1111j.1530-0277.2006.00085.x

Fisher, S. W. (2012). *The keeper: A novel.* Revell.
Gupta S, Warner J. Alcohol-Related Dementia: a 21st-century silent epidemic? *British Journal of Psychiatry* 2008;193: 351-353.

Harper C. The Neuropathology of alcohol-specific brain damage, or does alcohol damage the brain? *J Neuropathol Exp Neurol* 1998; 57:101-10.

Hazell AS, Butterworth RF. Hepatic encephalopathy: an update of pathophysiologic mechanisms. *Proc Soc Exp Biol Med.* 1999;222(2):99–112.

J Calderon, R J Perry, S W Erzinclioglu, G E Berrios, T R Dening, J R Hodges. Perception, attention, and working memory are disproportionately impaired in dementia with Lewy bodies compared with Alzheimer's disease. *J Neurol Neurosurg Psychiatry*, 2001;70:157–164.

Oslin DW, Streim JE, Parmelee P, Boyce AA, Katz IR: Alcohol abuse: a source of functional disability among residents of a VA nursing home. *Int J Geriatr Psychiatry* 1997, 12:825-832.

Ridley, NJ., Draper B, Withall A. Alcohol-related Dementia: and update of the evidence. *Alzheimer's Research & Therapy* 2013; 5:3.

Sechi GP, Serra A: Wernicke's encephalopathy: new clinical settings and recent advances in diagnosis and management. *Lancet Neurol* 2007, 6:442-455.

Sheedy D, Say M, Stevens J, Harper CG, Kril JJ. Influence of liver pathology on markers of postmortem brain tissue quality. *Alcohol Clin Exp Res*. 2012;36(1):55–60.10.1111/j.1530-0277.2011.01580.x

Thomson, A. D., Guerrini, I., & Marshall, E. J. (2012). The Evolution and Treatment of Korsakoff's Syndrome. *Neuropsychology Review, 22*(2), 81-92. doi:10.1007/s11065-012-9196-z.

Todd, K. G., & Butterworth, R. F. (1999). Mechanisms of Selective Neuronal Cell Death due to Thiamine Deficiency. *Annals of the New York Academy of Sciences, 893*(1 OXIDATIVE/ENE), 404-411. doi:10.1111/j.1749-6632.1999.tb07866.x.

Victor M, Adams RD, Collins GH. The Wernicke-Korsakoff syndrome: a clinical and pathological study of 245 patients, 82 with post-mortem examinations. *Contemp Neurol Ser* 1971; 7: 1–206.

Victor M, Adams RD, Cole M. The acquired (non-Wilsonian) type of chronic hepatocerebral degeneration. *Medicine. 1965; 44(5):345–396.*

Zaki AE, Wardle EN, Canalese J, Ede RJ, Williams R. Potential toxins of acute liver failure and their effects on blood-brain barrier permeability. *Experientia*. 1983; 39(9):988–991

Van Thiel DH, Gavaler JS, Tarter R, Schade RR, Stone BG. Hepatic encephalopathy and the neural regulation of hypothalamic pituitary function. *Semin Liver Dis*. 1985; 5(1):70– 83.10.1055/s-2008-104175.

Vetreno RP, Hall JM, Savage LM. Alcohol-related amnesia and dementia: Animal models have revealed the contributions of different etiological factors on neuropathology, neurochemical dysfunction and cognitive impairment. *Neurobio Learn Mem*, 2011; 96(4): 596-608.

5

THE APPREHENSION OF LIVING

> *"Living with fear stops us from taking risks, and if you don't go out on the branch, you're never going to get the best fruit."*
>
> — *SARAH PARISH*

Due to the trials and tribulations of my past life and family history, I have to be honest. I have endured a decade long battle with failed attempts at optimism and positivity regarding the future. I would typically experience immense stress when it came to predicting the minutes and days ahead. It was as if I was waiting for the sky to come crashing down upon my head.

For someone who has been through similar experiences

as I have, I would say that failure or disappointment are relatively normal expectations to have. Those who have led lives with minimal turbulence tend to remain upbeat, unable to detect the potential for disaster. One life event in particular has changed me so drastically that I believe I am forever different.

THE DAY THE GROUND DISAPPEARED BENEATH ME

It was a Friday mid to late October 2012, with two weeks past my first round of Psychology college exams, when I decided to visit my family for the weekend. Before leaving, I heard the whispers of a small snow storm, but nothing that seemed to draw my attention. I had no access to the news channel by choice, to put my studies first. Packing my laundry bags with my essential belongings, I had my parents pick me up from New Brunswick, NJ.

The weather was typical for the Bruns, windy and miserable. So I was happy to catch the scent of the ocean under my nose. We had a great time riding on the southbound parkway, listening to club music with my mom and brother. My dad decided to hold the fort down that night. We finally arrived in Seaside Park around 5 pm. I was so vibrant with excitement to be home, which seemed better than being trapped in the dormitory. We enjoyed the weekend together watching movies, our favorite shows, and chowing down on momma's famous home-cooked meals. The best part of them was sitting next to my dad on the couch with our puppy, Charlie. I appreciated that he was there to listen to how the past few weeks at college had been like for me. And somehow, no matter what I was worried about, he always managed to put me at ease.

As usual, my weekend of relaxation flew by. It was Sunday the 28th of Oct, time for me to return to college for classes later that night. As I was dreading doing so, there were a series of loud signals from the fire trucks outside. I didn't know what it was for until a fireman banged on our door saying that a massive storm was going to hit the island and we had to evacuate. My parents stood there in disbelief. To be honest, I almost did not believe that a storm of that magnitude would affect the island after the years of living here nothing like that had happened. But after turning the news on and looking at the predictions from the climatologists, we realized that it was not good. We thought we should protect ourselves, but we didn't know how. Realizing that the firemen were still outside, we asked them where we could go. The man said there are a number of shelters that are listed online in the neighboring town, Toms River.

I decided to take on the responsibility for rallying my apprehensive family together. This seemed to resemble the first time we were forced to pack our belongings and get out of dodge. My mom and dad were stubborn; they were not afraid of anything. They refused to be uncomfortable in a shelter with complete strangers for a night. As much as I understood their perspective, I had to disagree because our safety mattered most to me. What if an emergency happened, and we were the only ones stuck on the island? I argued this point to my family, and they started to take me more seriously. They finally seemed to comprehend what we were up against. Sure, we could survive the storm, but could we endure life without resources for weeks like in the aftermath of Hurricane Katrina?

Within the hour, I repacked my bags and put them in the trunk of our Chevy blazer, the truck that had pulled us through many emergency situations. Even though it broke down, here and there, we could always rely on it to keep running in times like this. After putting my stuff away, I helped my mom figure out what to bring for my dad and brother. She decided to make sandwiches, cook eggs, and bring all the snacks that we had. After all, we had no idea if we were even going to be fed or clothed. We thought we were simply just going to be there overnight or two at most. We had no way of knowing what was actually going to transpire.

We drove to one location in Toms River and it was at its maximum capacity. It seemed small for our taste given the storm we anticipated. So we drove hesitantly to the second location, Toms River High School North. This place was still accepting people in the shelter. They had a massive facility, and we were going to be staying in the gymnasium on cots. We filled out these forms for our family and then found our way over to our section. The volunteers grabbed our dog Charlie and put him in a cage in the back of the gym with the other animals, who spent most of the night whimpering and barking.

As I placed my laundry bag under my cot, I opened up the red cross blanket that was already sitting there for me. As the hours drew on, I noticed I was becoming feverish, and struggling to breathe properly. I didn't know what was happening, but it hit me like a ton of bricks. I heard there was a doctor on site so I went over to get checked out. I was told I was experiencing flu-like symptoms with respiratory distress. However, nothing could be done since they were not stocked with medication of that sort.

The night drew on as if it were daytime, since they never turned the lights out at the time one would expect. We heard the animals screaming, but the winds were howling louder. All of us in the room heard terrifying noises in the dead of night, leading us to be afraid of the damage we would wake up to. I barely slept, rolling around in the uncomfortable cot, feeling as sick as I could feel. And being forced to be around a whole gym full of people didn't help.

I remember waking up early in the morning to the local news crew coming in, to film all the people in the shelter. Apparently, on a few pieces of paper lay the fate of our houses. They started filming live reactions to the reactions of people whose homes were entirely destroyed by the water from the Atlantic Ocean meeting the bay. It was heartbreaking for me and my family. We received no news or updates about the condition of our house. From a moral standpoint, I found it entirely disrespectful and wrong for the news staff to force a microphone abruptly into everyone's faces just to provide the worst information possible. It was inconsiderate to wake everyone up at 5 am before being properly dressed or put together enough to receive information of that caliber. I struggled to breathe that morning because the concept of immense description felt like an elephant was sitting on my chest. I went back to my putrid green cot and covered myself with the white red cross blanket trying to hide from the pain of that morning.

When I awoke in search of caffeine, I began to feel psychologically manipulated by the fact that we had no access to TV or real news since that morning. Only police officers who had been on the island were disclosing information, but it was not much. I truly believe the individuals running the shelter were afraid to cause a mass panic among us. They suspected we would be fighting each other for resources and food. They were right. It would not take much to initiate chaos of epic proportions. I felt conflicted with emotions after coming to the conclusion that something was amiss.

In the case of a natural disaster, none of us knew what

to expect in that gymnasium. As if the individual bombs of news weren't enough, we were informed that the whole Seaside Heights boardwalk had been destroyed. The Ferris wheel where my first date took place was now sitting mangled in the ocean. The houses were displaced from their original locations and in the middle of the street. Speed boats were found crashed into houses and the sand covered the streets, making them impassable. Water was not yet retracting and dead animals were floating past the decrepit homes. Police officers and local heroes on boats and rafts were on rescue missions to find as many alive as possible. I don't know how my peers perceived this day, but this was the definition of a living nightmare. I began to believe that the world was coming to an end.

As the morning matured, the Red Cross was setting up tables with assigned case managers based on the letter or our last name. We were supposed to sign up for resources based on what we needed. So within the next 24 hours, more basic needs were delivered to us. Don't get me wrong, I was grateful for their efforts, but I still failed to comprehend the gravity of the damage that had been done. We had no service on our cell phones and no ability to see the news. We all struggled to come to terms with the fact that our home town was destroyed to the point where mostly everything needed to be rebuilt.

In my mind, I felt as though I had lost my home all over again but differently. The overall structure of our apartment was intact, but the bottom floor was damaged and in need of massive repair. There was no way that we would be able to move back in until we received a proper inspection and certificate of occupancy. I lacked the foresight at the time, to predict just how long we would be displaced for those repairs to take place. On the bright side, my family and I consider ourselves lucky; we made it out alive. Our home was damaged, but not beyond repair. I believe that a higher power was watching over us that day. My dog was not stranded like thousands of others that day, who perished waiting for rescue or suffered in fear, drowning to death.

It was barely a few days at this high school, before we were spontaneously forced to evacuate. A dozen yellow school buses pulled in out front of the gym waiting to pick us up. It seemed like we just became situated with the people and the environment, only to have our heads spinning all over again. We thankfully had our own vehicle and were able to follow the buses to an undisclosed location. Given the high stress of the situation, this trip made me so sick that we had to pull over so I could throw up on the side of the road.

When we approached the new shelter, I realized that we were going to be staying at Monmouth County Horse Race Track. The location was far from ideal, but happened to be the only location that was available to put all these stranded people. The walls were covered in this putrid white and forest green, while the floor looked like a maze of speckles. I had a feeling it wouldn't be long before I was sick of that place. My immediate thoughts were, where would all of us sleep? Apparently, there were cots set up in the main lobby all throughout the hallways, forced wherever they would fit so that the massive amount of stranded people could be accounted for until more permanent shelters were arranged for.

As my family and I settled in, I began to realize I was in close quarters with Seaside Heights hustlers and drug dealers. I witnessed drug deals left and right and the alcoholics suffering from withdrawals. I became concerned about my dad's sobriety. He was doing well at the time sticking to his proper diet and health care routine while still recovering from receiving Hepatitis C treatments months before. He was far from 100 %, but he was putting the work into improving his condition. Even accomplishing that would seem like a great feat for our family after the dozen times he had been in and out of rehab centers over the previous years. I was proud of him for taking accountability and turning our advice into action.

While walking around the racetrack, the scent of feces and urine clogged my nose and traversed the hallway next to the bathroom. Eventually, we wandered into the dining room and ate our first meal together as a family. It wasn't five-star quality food, but we were grateful to have any food given the circumstances. Later as I went to claim my cot, I realized that sleeping would be a task. We all had to rest with one eye open so that the dealers wouldn't steal our belongings for drugs. And trust me, there were parents showing their kids how to raid other people's cots for resources. The overall level of respect in that place just wasn't there. Because of that, I had nightmares when I did sleep and suffered from intense anxiety and fear.

We all tried to remain still, but the ground migrated beneath us. As a family, it took time to recover from being homeless for the first time. None of us were mentally prepared for moving to different places every few days because we could not return to our home. Technically, we were homeless again, but it was different this time. My father and mother felt particularly helpless since they were retired from work due to injury and disability. I felt like I had to be there for them this time, no matter what.

After a few days of being at this location, I had the opportunity to go back to my college dorm. So, I got a ride to New Brunswick from my boyfriend at the time. By a miracle I was able to get into contact with my family due to a hotspot internet connection. I was there for 2 days before I felt guilty. In fact, I was disgusted with myself for leaving my family stranded without my support. I found out they were transported again to Burlington County, New Jersey, essentially in the middle of farm lands. Filled with panic, I called a family friend and asked him for a ride to visit my family. I brought a bag with my only belongings because the dorm was still vacant for the most part. After my arrival, I saw my mom and dad thrilled just to have me there and I decided right then that I was not going to leave. So, I didn't. The consequence was losing the respect of my boyfriend, but that didn't matter to me. My family came first. I knew my mom, dad, and brother needed me by their side for comfort. There were no human beings on earth that could have destroyed the bond we shared.

At the time, I was simply relieved to be reunited. I was ready to endure any challenges, especially because I knew they were by my side. I could do anything as long as I had them. Another round of joy intermixed with relief set in when I heard that Charlie was transferred over to this facility and that I would be able to see him, unlike in the Monmouth County shelter. I was elated to embrace the dog that provided me with comfort on many sleepless nights.

In the Burlington shelter, we were finally able to settle in. After feeling like my own body odor was rotting my skin, we were awarded access to the washroom. Taking that first shower felt like heaven. It took the chill and achy feeling out of my bones for the first time since we evacuated. We had access to all the newly donated clothes, shoes, and jackets, allowing me to change into a clean outfit. The improvement in our living conditions provided all of us with a sense of hope that soon enough things would start to get better.

During that time, I was in my senior year at Rutgers University. The college was still closed because most of the state was stranded without power. Although school was a priority to me, it seemed secondary to what I was going through. I didn't believe that I could allow my family to suffer a second tragedy without me.

Weeks passed as power restoration was taking place. Slowly, people were able to get back on their feet, those who had been inland, anyway. Those of us from the island, still were wondering what would happen day to day. We had no official temporary housing until we could move back home. Little did we know how long that would actually take. After 3 more weeks in this shelter, case workers started meeting with people who needed to relocate. After all, the shelter was running low on resources to keep hundreds of people fed and clothed on a daily basis. We found out from being able to watch the news that the government had earned a grant or emergency fund to help all the people displaced from Superstorm Sandy. It felt like we were the last family to receive help. After all, relocation happened based on priority, those who were suffering from severe medical issues that needed access to additional resources and sleeping on cots were not conducive to accommodating disabled persons.

My memory of the situation regarding placing our family into temporary housing was a bit impaired. That may have been because I was not present for those conversations. Besides, even if I had access to hear the caseworker's suggestions, I was confident I would be terrified by all of them. No one wants to hear that they have to relocate because the government will only cover week to week stay in any form of temporary living residence, such as a hotel or bed-and-breakfast. Having to beg the government division, Federal Emergency Management Agency (FEMA), for money each week would be a great stress on us. I would hear my mother every few weeks on the phone asking who was going to cover the bill for the next few weeks. Because of this constant battle with state resources, I was mentally unequipped to process the daily stress. Little did I know, I had to. Hardening up would be the best thing for me. Would being insensate make the process easier? No, I didn't anticipate it would. But pretending was more preferable than acknowledging how much my heart pumped through my shirt, how I sweat out more calories than I was capable of consuming, and how much anger I managed to keep inside. These physical manifestations of stress seemed to become normal physiology for me. I often found myself going for a walk, in desperate search of a private spot, just so I could cry without an audience. I often felt robbed of that sacred moment of emotional catharsis, so it would continually accumulate until I felt like my organs were going to explode from the inside out. I truly believed the stress was taking a major toll on my body. And, even all these years later, there are the remnants of my ongoing battle with chronic stress. When I encountered mild stress, it caused a robust reaction. I began to devolve over time, since I was left unmanaged by coping skills, therapy, and psychotropic medications.

The next location I recall being drafted to was just off the boardwalk in Asbury Park, NJ. And when I tell you, it looked desolate, I'm pretty certain that would still lack the power to demonstrate how hopeless it felt to stay there. It apparently was the one beach town that had minimal damage because it was built higher than sea level. Even with the forty to fifty mile per hour winds, most structures maintained their integrity. Don't perceive my negative attitude as ungrateful. We were relieved to be out of cots for sure, but fitting four people in two beds was another thing. It just left privacy entirely out of the question. On the other hand, food became the next concern. The FEMA services only provided compensation for housing, which meant that we had to work day by day to combat starvation. Although the storm didn't kill us, it was entirely possible we would destroy each other by the end of this process.

Around this time, I had received news via email regarding campus re-openings. I was due to return and continue my classes.

Returning to school was one of the most dreaded decisions I had to make. Part of me wondered why I even went back after all that had happened. Because I had missed some classes due to receiving the email weeks after the fact, I was concerned I would not have the means to pass. Graduating would be nothing short of a miracle, especially given the fact that I was part of the Psychology Honors Program, which required that I write a senior thesis on a research experiment I conducted. When I arrived back into the laboratory, I was afforded some sympathy by the graduate student and undergrad staff. But after some time had passed, I was called into my mentor's office, since he was the principal investigator. As I walked down the hall, I could feel his sense of disdain contacting my energy field with strong bursts. When I sat down, I felt my stomach twisting like a towel caught in the washing machine. At first, he did not get right to the point. Then as if an airplane flew into my skull and blew my brains out the back of my head, he told me his brutal concerns. First of all, he didn't feel sorry for me enduring the storm. Because I had wasted so much time being there for my family, no work I could produce in a 2-month time span would be valuable. He told me I would not be worth taking a risk on, to ruin his solid reputation at the university. I walked out of that room speechless, feeling as worthless as a piece of garbage in a dumpster. I loathed myself for not having my research and data processed much sooner. If I had done more efficient work, we would not have had that conversation.

But I did what was necessary. I refused to give up. Of

course, it felt like 500 bees stung me in the chest; my pride was broken. Yet nothing would take away my determination to succeed and show this man that when I set my mind on a goal, there will be nothing stopping me.

It should be illegal to break someone's spirit. I never want to feel the way I felt walking out of his office that day, ever again. I do not feel it is beneficial in any way to put others down and ridicule them harshly. I cried and drank myself to sleep that night, and woke up the next day with a new head on my shoulders. I worked with the two graduate students in the lab to see if I could expedite my data analysis. The other concern was pulling my writing together. My advisor was right, the introduction section was a mess. Making the introduction and methods section, for the first time, required me to believe in myself. I was forced to take a close look at myself and realize that I am capable of so much. I have been the one holding myself back the whole time. It must have been all the self-doubts getting to my head. But this time, there was no choice. I was going to get my act together and complete this thesis no matter how much had to be sacrificed. I worked day and night, and even through to the morning to complete as much as possible. As I started sending my revised work to my professor, he was shocked. He did not expect the quality of work I provided. I truly gave it my all. Just because he started to believe in me again, that didn't mean I forgot what he said to me. I would never allow anyone to demean me in that same fashion ever again, not even if they think they're better than me, they are human too. I would love to see him walk a mile in my shoes.

After presenting my thesis and submitting the final copy, I was so relieved. My other thesis friends and I went out bar hopping. I was so burnt out tired by the end of this journey, that I looked forward to making things a blur. Over the next week, all the honors Psychology students waited for awards to be mentioned. What no one expected was that I would be included on that list. Not only did I win the award for best research project, I also won the most prestigious award that was offered, the Henry Rutgers Award. This award is for excellence as a leader, academic, and making a difference in the student community. I was so proud of myself for the first time. I have never done this work for recognition. I just wanted to do right by my professor and not embarrass the laboratory. I never imagined I would finish and produce high quality work, better than the other students. After this process, I realized I was more capable than I give myself credit for. If the Psychology department staff could recognize it, then how come I spent so long with my head down? Like I said, I believe it was related to the many years of bullying I endured had conditioned me to question myself. I never felt secure with my own abilities until that time. I learned a little lesson on how to pride myself, rather than create inner negativity.

What felt good at the end of my senior year was, being able to graduate, learning about my new found sense of confidence, making my parents proud, and most importantly, proving my mentor wrong. It felt so good to have him come and apologize to my face. I forgave him at that moment, but I have not forgotten the damage that believing in discouragement causes. I keep my sense of hope in my heart with me wherever I go to remind me of the moments where I lost it.

ADJUSTING TO A NEW NORMAL

That year took a lot out of me. I never expected the water to come and destroy our community, and I especially did not predict that my mentors would lose faith in me. After 6 months of my family moving between different hotels and shelters, we were finally able to move back to our apartment. There was still damage to the first-floor apartment, but the top floor, where we resided, had survived most of the impact. I relished in a sense of gratitude. It could have been much worse for us. But that is not to say that this experience was not emotionally draining in the least. I thank God and all the angels looking down on my family. I was grateful we decided to go to the shelter that day rather than ride the storm out alone, risking our ability to survive.

Despite the positives I drew from this situation, I

endured a few years of fear. I realized that my whole world could be turned upside down in an instant. That was what frightened me the most. I could have it all one day and the next day, be humbled to nothing. That is why I learned the importance of appreciating myself. That self-love I was a foreign concept to me. However, I needed to see my identity beyond the possibility of devastation and the negativity of doubt. After being homeless for the first time, I realized that I must love who I am. More importantly, I needed to learn to live without worrying about the world crashing down on me. Even if my life was comfortable and functional, I needed to be brave enough to risk losing it all. Beyond the adversity, I came to acquire immense strength. Look what I was able to overcome. It was by reframing my perspective that I was able to loosen the grip on my fear of living. No more being hesitant to live. I was only bound by the dimensions of my own mind. If I could adapt to each hurdle as a challenge, I would provide myself with a sense of reward, rather than defeat.

HOW TO TAKE BACK THE CONTROL OF YOUR LIFE

- Realize that you cannot control all circumstances that affect you or the people around you. You can only control your own behavior.
- Use your fears as motivation to keep going. We all have fears, but it is how we respond to them that makes the difference. This means, do not give up at the slightest hurdle, doubt, or discouragement from others. Just because we are uncertain of what may happen, this doesn't mean you should stop trying.
- Fight for yourself when no one else will. There will be many occasions when the people around you work hard to prevent you from being successful. Take their behavior with a grain of salt. Do not hesitate to unleash your full potential. Draw on your past failures and setbacks for answers. From this you can obtain the wisdom to proceed in accomplishing your goals.
- When you face rejection and criticism, remain patient. Other positive opportunities will arise. Sometimes we need to be rejected to motivate us to keep reaching for the better outcomes we deserve.

- Do not give up, no matter what! No matter how bad things get, do not stop trying to become your best self. Nothing in the world is worth giving up on yourself for. Even if you are left mentally defeated, process the setback as a learning experience and try again.

References

Sarah Parish Quotes. (n.d.). https://www.brainyquote.com/quotes/sarah_parish_570764

6

THE UNCERTAINTY OF SUCCESS

> *"Our deepest fear is not that we are inadequate, it is that we are more powerful beyond measure. It is our light, not our darkness that frightens us. We ask ourselves, who am I to be brilliant, gorgeous, talented, fabulous? Actually, who are you not to be?"*
>
> — *MARIANNE WILLIAMSON.*

As a child, I struggled to believe that I could become successful following any of my dreams. No matter what my goals were, feelings of self-doubt plagued me. Looking back, I believe I lacked confidence because of the learning disabilities I faced as a child.

When I was born on October 1st, 1991, I was a premature baby. Because of this, I struggled with learning. A particular challenge for me was understanding mathematics and numbers. For some reason, that part of my brain early on failed to conceptualize the intention and application of this subject. Over the first few years of my life, my mom began to realize that it was difficult to capture my attention with. At one point, she was concerned that I was deaf. So, she took me to the doctor, and it turned out that I needed glasses and was one tone short of needing a hearing aid. Even though it might not seem significant, the first 3 years before this was discovered impaired my ability to comprehend material in preschool. Although I was hungry to grow up and be independent, I needed to learn differently than the other students. However, by the time I was exposed to more complicated concepts in elementary school, I had trouble with most teaching styles. For many years, I had no idea what my style of learning should be. By the time I reached the 3rd and 4th grade, I was in special education. Yes, this is the portion of the day where students are taken out of class for extra assistance. This is to help guide slow learners by using additional teacher resources.

The only subject I was good at was English. I especially enjoyed creative writing and poetry. Writing allowed me to express myself in ways that I never could verbally. I would become easily embarrassed because I would stutter on my words when I tried to speak. And so, that's what made me shy and uncomfortable. After Special-Ed each day, I would return to class, hide behind my glasses, and hold my head down in shame. That became my journal time, where I would avoid conversation at all costs. The kids in this upper-class town were snobby and judgmental, especially if I didn't wear designer clothes. I appreciated my parents' hard work to raise me and I didn't deserve to be criticized for not being rich enough.

Most often, this journal time was used to describe my feelings regarding others and the way they mistreated me. I was disappointed that no one could look past my lenses to see that I had this big heart. I was picked on, like I had mentioned earlier just because I was perceived as meek and powerless compared to the other kids at school. Real people would pull my hair, beat me up, and throw rocks in my face. I just did not have the time for it. So, my journal became my best friend that comforted me when I was terrified to be myself. I told the aqua blue pages of my unicorn studded journal what my dreams were, who I had a crush on, and all my secrets.

For quite some time, academics remained a problem for me. It took years before I was able to overcome my trouble learning.

In early elementary school, I found yet another outlet for my frustrations. I discovered my blossoming relationship with music. Every time I heard a song I loved on the radio; my energy lightened. I would make it my business to learn all the words so I could sing along. This unrelenting passion for music eventually developed into dancing and acting.

I still remember my early interactions with music. In the beginning, I would listen to music over kids' movies. My mom always said that I was awestruck every time I interacted with music. In order to develop my skills with music, she signed me up for ballet. I recall being so proud to show my mother the grace and elegance I learned in my first show. I am grateful to my mother for providing me with this opportunity because it taught me mental discipline. As I look back to that moment, I can feel her watching me, being so proud that her eyes glimmered from the audience.

As a preteen, dancing became means for expressing my stagnant and negative emotions. I could stand out without having to speak or be singled out for being different. In our ballerina uniforms we were all the same. The few years between ages 7 and 10, the need to dance transformed into the desire to become a singer and actress. I was comforted by the fact that music could temporarily cure my pain and manage my emotions. Each time I would sing and dance my heart out, the negative energy dissipated. I created a protective barrier of goodness between myself and others. For the first time, I gained my independence and embraced my skills as an individual, rather than comparing myself to others. I was beginning to be happy with being me. Maybe being myself wasn't so bad after all.

My first mentor made a huge impact on my life. He was one of my neighbors down the street from our Westfield home. He first developed a comradery with my mother. He owned a photography studio and photo printing center known as *Photofinish*. Now this was the era before digital when film was brought to a store to be developed. It was a great place that I personally spent a lot of time at since my mom was learning how to become a photographer. Moreover, he was a figure in the Westfield and Kenilworth, and NJ communities, working with local police departments and theatre companies to develop their photos. He had me audition for the first theatrical performance, *Annie*. Let me just say that I had no idea what I was doing in terms of how to present myself. At that point, I had training in dance, but had little to no official experience with live singing. He took me aside, for as long as it required, to teach me how to sing from my 'gut' a.k.a., diaphragm. Because of him, I learned how to control my breathing to create the appropriate pitches and note intensity. He refused to give up on me, even when I had those moments where I couldn't hit the right note and would start crying as a result of giving up on myself. More importantly, I learned to remain in character while doing so. If the show required singing with an accent, I was taught to remain consistent with it. It was the first time in my life I was trained in all three disciplines. I thought that maybe one day I could be a triple threat.

Despite these wonderful experiences, I struggled to feel good enough. This is probably because I would compare myself to others and automatically feel Inferior. I saw their lack of fear and it bothered me that I couldn't be just like those other girls, who landed leading roles. After a while, I began to question whether I was good enough to even participate in public theatre. I genuinely believe this low self-esteem emerges from the daily embarrassment I faced in Special Education. I always thought I was far behind everyone else.

By the time I neared the end of fourth grade, I met one of my good friends to this day whose mother was opening a local modeling and talent agency. I was lucky enough to not only receive a letter in the mail but also work there to help get the business up and running. I was beyond ecstatic to have the opportunity to go on auditions and open calls. And that is exactly what I had the opportunity to do. As I spent time getting to know her, I realized she was truly a great friend. With her long red, curly hair and freckles, she has this sense of humor that bordered on inappropriate sarcasm. Although she crossed the line sometimes with her humor, this is what I love most about her. She was one of the few girls I was able to be vulnerable with and trust to share my deepest secrets with. And in return, I learned to become a good listener. She even took me to places I had never been before.

I can remember one of our beach visits vividly. The sun was strong but in a good kind of way, not the need to pass out from the humidity. I could smell the sea air rush under my nostrils and the sun rays permeate the outer layer of my skin. It was as if we were together against the world on this majestic beach. The sun was so strong that it sparkled off the sand and water, lacing it with glitter.

That day, she and I believed this place existed for the purpose of our exploration. We casually walked across the black asphalt with our thin flip flops on, approaching the beach with a sense of childish merriment. We took off our shoes and our feet mingled with the sand. I laid my towel down next to hers with a sense of jittery excitement for the day ahead.

The one thing that made this day special was that I felt so comfortable around her family. I have never felt this with any of my previous friends' parents. There was always some kind of cultural or race difference that was harped upon, created to make me feel as though I were an inferior. I never looked at anyone different from me with a sense of distaste or disgust. I saw the good in people regardless of their outward appearance. To this day, I am entirely grateful to her parents for being such good people and treating me like her own child. To her mother, looking down on me from heaven, thank you for being there to support my dreams.

After relaxing with my feet in the sand, she and I decided to get up and go to the ocean water to cool off. It was always important to warm up in the hot sand first before doing so, almost customary. The water was perfect and so was our time together. She never let me down, always genuine and straightforward, and never snobby from living on the upper-class side of town. Our family, on the other hand, was lower middle class. She never saw that when she looked at me. I was never less than according to her. I still appreciate what she has done for me even today. After coming out of the water and returning to the towel, we decided to go to the amusement section at the boardwalk. We went on as many rides as we could.

Having my best friend and her mother by my side, I began to believe that good things could be possible.

It was not too long after spending time with their family that I was invited to go on auditions. My mom was so proud of me, I remember her unrelenting excitement. She took me to a family friend to get headshots taken. After that, we were in and out of New York City. I was invited to be an extra on the set of several movies such as *Spiderman 2*, *Then She Found Me*, and *Raising Helen*, and tried out for a few commercials. I did meet a few shining stars along the way. The one concept that struck me was that famous people are not superheroes, they are real humans. I guess it is one of those thoughts that cannot be conceptualized until you are standing in front of one. You come to notice why they receive the attention they do, then the other part of you feels sorry that they are robbed of a normal life. Even so, I still have always wanted this. And although not having enough money has delayed this journey at times, my friend and her mother reminded me to never give up.

With persistent determination and little confidence, I started to develop my skills by writing song lyrics. These words became the translation of my soul's mirror. All those lyrics still represent parts of who I am today. What makes me feel organically connected to sounds and tunes are the vibrations that are emitted which change my vibe instantly. For some reason, I was born with the ability to feel emotions and music in the form of physical energy. If I were around pessimistic people, I would search for a song that would oppose the darkness. I deserved those moments of peace, for I lacked the ability to understand the concept of happiness. That was a direct result of not being educated or exposed to the appropriate coping skills for a maturing adolescent. I had no idea what I was supposed to do to make improvements in myself mentally. As a result, I would work on singing higher notes, writing better songs. I started off slow as most would before learning to record and produce my own music.

QUIET THE NOISE OF DOUBT

Looking back, I realize how much talent I had. I often wonder how it is possible that I am not famous. I now believe that I was my own worst enemy. I was terrified to put myself out there. In fact, I would freeze up when it came time to show what I was made of. Reflecting on this time bothers me. And it's all because I worried so much about what other people thought of me. In reality, I should not have lived my life in fear of being disliked by others. That anxiety became so strong that it prevented me from trying at all most of the time. If I could tell my readers one thing only, it would be to start living for you and no one else. People can share their opinions, but at the end of the day, it does not reflect who you truly are. For example, someone can say you are ugly, but that is just how they perceive you. Opinions are useless because they reflect nothing of the truth. Therefore, I encourage you to live your life placing no value on what other people think.

Secondly, I would advise you to stop questioning everything about yourself. I always had this ability to question everything. The problem is I drove myself nuts. Maybe this was a consequence of depression, but being filled with uncertainty makes me succumb to the negativity rather than remaining positive.

I have been reframing the way my mind constructed thoughts over the past year. No one will ever know the way each individual talks to themselves. That is a good thing, because if we heard those self-criticisms, we would agree that they are unbelievably harsh. I realized that if I wanted to identify the frequency and volume of these thoughts, I must make a record of them. To my surprise, putting them on paper has been the biggest relief.

In the field of Psychology, the processes that perpetuate negativity are known as *maladaptive cognitions*. So how did I learn to recognize them within myself? I would not be able to take all the credit for this, even though I have taken responsibility for all of my problematic behaviors. I had a great support system when I reached out for help with my depression, anxiety, PTSD, and substance dependency. I had taken those thoughts so far to the point of planning my own death and taking the steps to carry it out. I would self-medicate, using anything that would prevent me from crying or from inflicting self-harm and my anger accruing into more severe forms of punishment.

During the process of disentangling my whole emotional system and examining my flaws piece by piece, I made a list of the way I would talk to myself. In the beginning, I failed to recognize that they were detrimental to my mental health. But after writing them down, I was instructed to write the positive version of those thoughts on the other side of the paper. Before following the task, I added to the exercise by adding a middle step of neutral cognitions. For me, it was much easier to become neutral before being positive due to my struggles with depression. Eventually, those poisonous self-criticisms were no longer swirling through my bloodstream, preventing me from appreciating my true self. I am grateful for this lesson because I never realized just how much I prevented my own success. I would be so close to the apex of my career and just never reach it. And honestly, I have myself to blame. Just performing a simple task, I could see the dichotomy between myself and the normal people surrounding me.

Here's an example of what my paper looked like:

Current Cognitions

- I am not worthy of happiness.
- I will never amount to anything.
- I am too skinny to be loved.
- I'll never be good enough.
- I am a failure.
- Nothing will ever get better for me.
- I look like the girl that no one wants to be friends with.
- I'm a has been.
- I will be in an unhealthy relationship, as long as I'm alive. This is because I have had communication issues with my father.

Neutral Cognitions

- I am not a success, but I am not exactly a failure. I am just an average human being trying to make it in the world.
- I don't know if things will get better, but I can only hope.
- Success in life is not exponential, just because I am not where I want to be doesn't mean that I can't work for it.

Ideal Cognitions

- I am worthy of happiness.
- I am good enough.
- I love myself no matter what people say.
- Yes, I am a thin girl, but there is someone out there to love me.
- I am not a failure.
- Things will get better for me.
- I am who I am now and there's nothing wrong with me.
- I will be in a healthy relationship one day as long as I can properly address the issues with my father.

I realized as a result of these internalized negative

thoughts; I had become inherently perfectionistic. Nothing I did was ever good enough. Any final copy would always be a work in progress. In my mind, there was always more that I can do. In order to address these thoughts, I would also need to compromise on my need to be flawless with everything, and especially my need to be so hard on myself. So how would I even begin to improve? Part of recovering the beautiful, uncriticized parts of myself would require me spending time with others who also share similar flaws. I started to attend group therapy. And some of those exercises required all of us to write something nice about each person in the room anonymously, even if we didn't know them. This seems stupid, and, of course I thought it was lame, but it forced me for a moment to look for the positive qualities in others. This was the first step. It allowed me to see that if someone can meet me for the first time and find something heartwarming and complimentary to say, why can't I, after knowing myself for all these years? Exactly. I didn't love myself the way I should. I focused on what I wasn't good at and all of my flaws, rather than my assets. Part of this can be attributed to my traumatic life experiences - always seeing the glass half empty trained my expectations to be negative. I realized that I have been the one that held myself back from success for so many years.

There is no easy formula to fixing your entire life, but there is a way to do so. This requires changing your mindset. If I did not take the time to change the way I perceived my life, there would have been no growth. So, as you take this journey along with me to visit my fears, I hope that you can learn to make improvements in your own life.

HOW TO EMBRACE & FOSTER SUCCESS

Understand that you cannot be perfect. It is okay to let your imperfections shine. They become lessons that help us grow. If you're penalized for your mistakes, let it roll off your back. I've discovered that it is probably because they are fundamentally unhappy with their own abilities. In return, they criticize the people around them to make themselves feel better.

Find your passion, because that becomes a positive outlet. For me, music became my way of expressing my negative emotions. It took me out of my anger during difficult moments. If you have some activity that does that for you, I encourage you to continue to follow that. Most of the time doing what you love is what will boost your success. This is because you become less resentful towards others, being free to follow your passion, instead of being stuck at a job you hate.

Make your goals realistic & obtainable. If you expect to have all your goals accomplished overnight, that just is not possible. Goals should be small building blocks that slowly bring you to the final goal. If you try to do too much in a small period of time, you risk disappointment and even failure.

Do NOT GIVE UP ON YOUR DREAMS! There are so many people who are going to hate on you along the way, or try to discourage you from pursuing your dreams. But I am here to tell you to ignore what people say. Sometimes the people around us are so stuck in their miserable lives that they see no way out. And so, when they look at you, they react with pessimism. You must stay focused on your dreams regardless of judgements from others. I am here to remind you to never give up, no matter how many challenges you face. It will make it much more worth it in the end. If I listened to all the people that doubted me, I would not be where I am today.

Change your Cognitions. Embracing your success requires you to work on changing your thoughts. You cannot achieve your dreams if you continue to talk to yourself in a negative manner. You do not want to end up being your own worst enemy.

References

Grady, C. (2019, July 30). Why Marianne Williamson's most famous passage keeps getting cited as a Nelson Mandela quote. https://www.vox.com/culture/2019/7/30/20699833/marianne-williamson-our-deepest-fear-nelson-mandela-return-to-love

7

INTIMIDATION OF INSANITY

"Lose your mind and come to your senses"

— *FRITZ PERIS*

During my late 20s, I had experienced severe emotional issues. It's important for me to address the elephant in this book and the secondary motivation for sharing my story. This is the part of my life that caused me to have a serious mental breakdown prior to reaching out for help. For every waking moment, I would suffer with flashbacks of the painful memories of my past. I was never truly unencumbered by the traumas of my past. So, when these last two events occurred, it drove me to the edge of ending my own life. In the moments prior to this breakdown, I would be alive, but never living in the current moment. I would see a dad with his daughter and remember the loss of my own. I missed the bond I used to have. And each of those daily interactions would serve as a trigger for my panic. The more I tried to fight it, the more it made me sick. Just the thought of consuming food made my stomach churn. Sleeping was by far the worst. I jostled around in the bed like there were fire ants in the covers, constantly awakened by the feeling of being choked. The only way time my brain would try to resolve my own dilemmas, solutions, and fears was in my sleep. Some of my worst fears matured into intense dramatizations of reality that challenged my psyche. For the most part, I was not ready to protect myself against them.

Prior to my admittance to the mental hospital, I had two major life-changing events that sent me over the edge. It is important for me to talk about these events because they have become a catalyst for, not only my downward spiral, but also the reason for my recent success.

One morning, I was sleeping as I had not in weeks. I happened to be in my mother's room, falling asleep from the movie we both watched the night before. As I laid, I was startled by the sensation of a strange panting sound that was so unusual, it woke me up. Because this sound was not part of the typical range of morning noises my mom made, my senses told me something was wrong. Her discomfort radiated into vibrations that caused chills upon my whole body. I jumped up like there was a fire in the bed and took a look at my mom. It was at this very moment that my senses became aware, like a wolf focusing on its prey in the darkness.

I jolted towards her to examine her body language. All my mental evaluations of her past behavior now told me that she was far from her normal alert condition. As I inspected her from top to bottom, I realized she was sweating profusely by the way her little stray hairs stuck to her face. She was experiencing difficulty breathing and this became apparent by the way she was becoming increasingly unresponsive to me. In normal circumstances, this would not be alarming if this were summer and my mom had just finished doing laundry. However, since it was winter, all I could think was that I needed to find my phone and call 911. Something was seriously wrong. I knew in my heart. I panicked that every wasted second could count against me. Not everyone survives their first scrape with death.

I acted quickly by finding the nearest phone. Immediately, I dialed the three numbers, but I became frustrated because the service was terrible. I am surprised they heard what I was saying because of the poor signal along with my slurred speech from the intense panic inside me. This almost prevented my ability to form words. When the first responder responded, I could barely breathe. I fail to recall what I said because in those moments since I was in a daze, but I did what I could to help her remain conscious.

I was in such shock that every word that came out of my mouth felt like it was coming from someone else. It was hard for me to process what was happening. I couldn't even believe the fact that my mom was in that condition, unable to communicate with me. I was almost certain that I would be losing her. This was my only surviving parent and I could not handle losing her. They 911 operators urged me to remain calm, so I stayed on the phone with them until the ambulance showed up.

By this point, I picked my mom up and brought her from her bedroom to the couch so she could be assessed and transported out of the apartment easier. But when the EMTs arrived, I was in for another shock. They were the most unprepared and ill-trained "professionals" I had ever seen.

When they first arrived, they asked if my mom consumed any drugs. They first suspected she was having an overdose. First of all, that was the wrong assumption to make. Just because many others in town have suffered this same fate, doesn't mean it is also happening here. This made me angry because these crucial minutes were wasted on questions instead of stabilizing her vitals.

After explaining to them that drugs were not the problem, they continued their half-assed attempt at checking her. I made the statement that I believed she was having a heart attack because her chest was hurting. As I said this, she began to lose consciousness completely. At that moment, my world stood still. I froze in shock begging her to stay with me. I saw she was on the edge and I wanted to give her a reason to fight.

Adding to the stress of the situation, they brought an oxygen tank that did not work. I believe that this is why she passed out entirely. So it was quite some time she had been without a proper air supply. Had they brought one that functioned properly to start with, she might not have been unconscious. In my mind, my anger was multiplying into rage and extreme anxiety. I was at this point, in a full body tremble that made my mouth chatter as I tried to speak.

As this fiasco continued, I begged God to not take my mother from me. I just could not handle it. Plus, I would not be okay with losing her due to a medical mistake. Finally, within another minute, they asked one member of the response team via radio to bring another one up the stairs. When that was strapped to her face, they failed to turn it on. My thoughts at this moment were who allowed these individuals to become emergency responders. Their mistakes could have cost me my mother. And that is something, I knew would mentally break me. Just even the threat of it sent me in a tailspin, so I cannot imagine the situation turning out worse.

Despite the chaos of the morning, I am grateful to God

that he put me there to be by her side. I truly believe that if I had called even one moment later, she would have been gone. She would not have been able to endure another ten minutes of struggling to breathe. When the ambulance transported her down the stairs, they got her into the ambulance and rushed her to the nearest hospital.

She was given an EKG to look at her heart. The doctor said she had a major heart attack due to one hundred percent blockage of the carotid artery. She also had approximately 70 percent blockage in the other two main arteries. The doctors said it was a miracle she survived, because most people don't live through that kind of heart attack. In order to keep her heart beating, doctors put a stent in to clear her carotid artery and restore blood flow.

Despite the fact that my mom survived, everything inside me changed. I struggled to speak about my feelings. I held them in and tried my best to remain strong for her and my brother. But deep down, I was breaking down emotionally. During the time my mom remained in the hospital for observation, I returned down that dark road of drinking and self-medicating. I could not handle any more grief and near-death experiences. I was terrified that something would happen to her again if I were not watching her. This led to a nagging feeling of self-induced guilt whenever I failed to do enough for her.

Her several days in the Intensive Care Unit forced me to consider that it would be just my brother and I one day.

Just thinking about it took the breath out of my lungs. How would I fare mentally with her gone? Of course, I am a strong-willed woman, but I was not equipped to live without her. I needed at least one parent to be there for the birth of my first kid and my wedding. I needed her to be proud of me when I did the right things, and to kick me in gear when I get off track.

We have always been accountable for each other. Without her to counterbalance my moments of irresponsibility, I feared being alone and falling off into a dark abyss where no one could pull me out. And my brother would be worse off without her. He still had so much to learn.

From that moment forward, everything in my life changed. Not only was I a different person, but so was my mom. She could no longer be the same woman that could do it all. It is not as though she didn't try, but with stents in her chest, her abilities became limited. She could no longer exert herself the way that she used to. This meant that our activities together would no longer be the same.

I knew that from then on, I would need to put forth more effort into helping take care of her. It seemed like not that long ago when everything was fine and nothing would stop her from taking on the world. I guess part of growing up is realizing that our parents are not going to remain in perfect health forever. If I saved face and did not tell anyone how bad I was hurting, I believed it would go away. But instead, the nightmares became worse, I almost never slept, and eating was an even bigger challenge. I was desperately consuming any substances that eased my pain and helped me to feel better on the momentary basis. It has taken me a long time to admit this because I am ashamed that I took on the same qualities of my father - not communicating, and just dosing myself into a deep sleep where none of the daytime torture can reach me.

It took me a few months of maladjustment to calm down enough to return to some kind of mental and physical normalcy. I finally got back to sleeping more regularly, eating, and going back to work without having to leave. At this time, my brother was seeing an older woman (for privacy purposes, I shall not mention her name). She seemed to be in love with him, and I know he was in love with her. I just failed to see how things would progress over the course of a few months after my mom's heart attack. She seemed nice enough at first. Then she came to live with us, without my mom's permission. She had indicated that her daughter was arguing with her, had cleared her bank account, and kicked her out the house. This left her nowhere to go. From my point of view, she had an odd personality. She seemed like a cat that is skittish of people. She had blonde hair and piercing light blue eyes that had this indifference about them. I never saw her truly excited, but I could see something dark behind those eyes that I just couldn't explain. I chalked this up to maybe she was intimidated or uncertain of my mom and I, because she was in her late forties and my brother in his late twenties. So, I could easily see how this may be difficult for her to approach my mom and I freely, without any hesitations.

After staying with us for quite some time, my mother and I noticed that she was slowly bringing more and more of her stuff. Just being nice, my mom didn't want to tell her to leave. So, with some qualms, we allowed her to move in because we are just not the kind of family that kicks someone when they're down, especially given the experiences that we have faced together with homelessness. Early on, she was quite difficult to speak with, other than the usual non-verbal acknowledgement of our existence. We just thought she was shy. But then she started to speak more to my mom and I and we began to develop a relationship with her. I began to become angry with myself for not giving her a chance. I thought my brother had to love her for a reason, so maybe my instincts were wrong about her. However, I knew in my heart they would not last together. Plus, they had so little in common and were at two different ends of life.

It took several months to encourage her to speak more freely to my mother and I. Her shyness was fading and we started to feel like our family was whole again for the first time since my dad's death. So, thanksgiving rolled around and we planned on cooking a turkey. Since she had not cooked in a while, she offered to help my mother to keep her busy. The dinner turned out nice and my mother and I both fell into a post turkey coma with the smell still lingering throughout the apartment. It wasn't long before I was asleep. In fact, it must have only been minutes before I entered a dream state.

As I was finally relaxing, my brother ran into the room with a sense of urgency. His eyes were wide with tears and he was struggling to get the words out. He said that his girlfriend was unresponsive, turning blue, and urinating herself. My mom and I jumped up out of bed rapidly to check on her. Based on those symptoms, the cause of her current condition was perplexing.

When I opened my brother's bedroom door, I realized how bad the situation was. I found her unconscious, making animalistic grunting noises. The piercing sound of her choking on her own saliva was permanently imprinted in my mind. With my previous experience working in a laboratory with mice, I was familiar with heart-palpitating death gasps. I had little time to react before losing her entirely, so I ran and grabbed the phone and immediately called the emergency services. I described her strange symptoms. It took what felt like an eternity for them to arrive, and this is probably because it was around 2 in the morning.

While remaining on the phone with emergency operators, I grabbed his girlfriend in my arms, dragging her carefully off the bed. I properly positioned myself on the floor to brace her limp weight. I held her upright to make sure she wasn't choking on her own saliva. Holding her with one arm and the phone against my neck, I pushed on her chest hoping it would help her breathe. If knew if she remained laying down, she might not have survived. I kept going, and for a moment, it seemed like she was starting to breathe again. But she wasn't. She was barely hanging on by a thread. After continuing to rub her chest and keep her top half upright, I noticed that she was starting to come back a little. I was slightly relieved but still in immense panic because I knew she would not make it very long without medical assistance.

It wasn't too much later that the EMTs arrived. A flock of seven or eight of them showed up. Sadly, their actions mirrored that morning my mom had the heart attack. They tried to work on her from my brother's bedroom floor, but they were in a cramped space. Not long after, they transported her to the couch on the right side of our apartment. During this time, they were all poking, prodding, and trying to get vitals from her. At this time, their primary concern was her blood pressure was so high that when they tried to put an oxygen mask on her, real blood started squirting out towards me seven feet away. At that point, I became disturbed by the way they stood there stupefied and uncertain of what to do. They brought various pieces of tubing, masks, radios and left them spread out over our apartment without putting them to use.

For quite some time, the EMTs were uncertain of the

cause of her current condition. She was writhing, making animalistic grunting noises. It was as if she were no longer human at that moment. Certainly, I could no longer recognize the real her in any of her curious behaviors.

As she was fighting to stay alive, I became increasingly concerned about the welfare of my brother and my mom. I saw my mom standing on the side holding her chest in pain. I was worried that this situation would send my mom back to the hospital with another heart attack. She stood in the corner holding her chest with my brother on the other side of her sobbing in pain. We all thought for sure she would not make it, but by some miracle she held on just long enough to get her to the hospital for evaluation. In those moments, I have to believe that there are angels protecting me and my loved ones from the other side. Besides, how else would these kinds of miracles happen?

We followed the ambulance to the hospital and waited for her to get set up in the emergency room. When we arrived, I noticed she was looking at us as if she no longer recognized us. So, I asked her who I was and she was not sure. Then I pointed to my brother and mom, and her response was the same. With each failed identification, my concern grew. I reminded her who I was and that my brother and mom were there. Rather than acknowledging us, she continued to ask repeatedly what was happening. This was not a normal phrase that would come out of her mouth from day-to-day conversation. Even worse, I noticed that her pupils were unusually large and she didn't improve within the half an hour we had been there. The doctor told us she had a seizure and that she would be out of it for a little while before returning to her normal condition. Ten to fifteen minutes after, she wasn't showing signs of improvement.

Because the doctors were not acting quickly enough, I decided to follow what my own training in Neuroscience taught me from Rutgers University. Pupil dilation was a general indicator of bleeding in the brain. Plus, her inability to address us by name or recognize our presence was a sign of internal brain bleeding. She never hit her head, but it didn't mean bleeding was impossible. Because of her ongoing confusion, I urged the nurses to perform a CT scan. I explained to her my expertise in studying the brain from Rutgers and she knew that what I was saying was right. Besides, it couldn't hurt to check. Her blood pressure prior to arrival was very high. That was enough to cause all the vessels in the brain to burst. I was quite surprised that these signals were ignored and she was going to be sent home had I not spoken up.

Even after knowing my brother's girlfriend for only a year, I cared for her and she became part of our family. They finally wheeled her down the hall for the brain scan. Within ten to fifteen minutes, the nurse and doctor came running into the emergency room saying there was massive bleeding in the right side of the brain. The next best decision would be to airlift her to Robert Wood Johnson in New Brunswick, NJ where the best and most practiced Neurosurgeons in the state exist. I was proud they were going to be taking her to the hospital where my aunt and Uncle practice medicine. Moreso, I was proud to have received an education from the same school. If it were not for my extensive learning and taking advanced courses in Neuropsychology, I would not have seen the signs of her trouble.

She survived the airlift, but she was so far from being out of the woods. To everyone's dismay, the source of internal bleeding was difficult to isolate, even after taking more additional high-resolution scans. First, the doctors performed a procedure to clamp the bleeding so they could drain the rest of the fluid out without increasing intracranial pressure. After doing so, there was still a small leak. Two more procedures later, they were able to temporarily clamp the region that was inflicting the most damage. For the most part, this is what kept her alive. However, the surgeons made it very clear that that was not the end all solution; massive brain surgery was still required to stop the bleeding with one hundred percent certainty and make sure the rest of the fluid was cleaned out. Moreso, they wanted to install a more permanent clamp with an internal drain. This would manage and prevent small bouts of bleeding throughout her life.

These doctors were my heroes. Having the experience

performing cannula implantation in mice brains, it is not an easy task. I will forever praise them for saving her life. Most people who endure aneurysms do not survive, nevermind make it through several procedures.

HOW BRAIN SURGERY IMPACTED HER EMOTIONAL PROCESSING

An unfortunate consequence of her brain surgery was an inability to understand emotion from others in the same way. She became egocentric, only worrying about her own issues. When members of our household had something important to do, she would throw tantrums demanding that her needs come first. And even worse, she became increasingly aggressive, which was probably a result of the residual bleeding affecting the systems controlling her emotional regulation. She began to refuse help from the hospital staff and became aggressive when they would ask for her cooperation. This was a stark difference from how she was before the aneurysm. It made improvements in her recovery a struggle at best. Getting her to work on her speech and physical therapy posed many challenges, given her overall lack of motivation. She lost the ability to believe in herself and certainly became paranoid of the intentions of others.

For my brother, this event traumatized him greatly. To add insult to injury, she made him feel guilty for not doing enough for her on a regular basis. In reality, he spent the majority of his daily income on her to help her survive. Her personality seemed to change for the worse. She began to believe that we were all against her and she would refuse to communicate with my mother and I, even though we waited on her hand and foot. The major consequence was that our family dynamics were permanently altered. She no longer listened to or comforted him, and refused to be a participant in her own self-care. Even worse, she failed to be a useful contributing member of the household despite being physically functional.

MY EMOTIONAL TRANSFORMATION POST-TRAUMA

Because of these situations, I started to hit a mental rock bottom. I developed a complete distrust in my faith and no longer believed that a good life was possible. As a result, my self-medicating worsened. To make matters worse, I became involved with the wrong crowd of people. The addiction fueled environment perpetuated my downward spiral. Constantly being surrounded by a town full of people with mental and emotional issues only exacerbated mine. I was not sure how to tell myself that everything would be alright. Nearly losing my mom and the situation with my brother's girlfriend caused me to lose my own ability to take care of myself. This led me to want the darkest place I've ever been - suicide. I wanted to be dead, and I tried to take too many drugs to take my own life.

There was no more believing that everything would be alright. Hope and optimism were replaced by hopelessness and anger. I never imagined that I could surpass the pain or forgive God for trying to take away what's left of my family. I mean how much more could He take? I spent months unable to sleep, sick to my stomach. And when I looked in the mirror, there was nothing left but a shell of a person. My soul was dissipating through the scars of my pain. The dark circles under my eyes looked worse against a backdrop of skin and bones. I never imagined that I could recover or gather the proper coping skills to live a normal life again. I starved myself because food no longer brought me any comfort. In fact, the thought of a meal made me sick because of the amount of tension that remained in my body.

As each day went by, I began to wonder how reparation could begin. I was so lost that I was sure nothing could find me. I believed I might never find the strength within myself.

Because of this experience, I have learned so much. So, I have dedicated the next chapter to showing how my will to die showed me how to live. I hope you can find inspiration from knowing that you are not alone in your struggles, feelings of hopelessness, and suicidal thoughts. Give me a chance to show you why I realized life is worth living before making any rash decisions. Even though it may seem though your life is over, it isn't. I can only tell you this as a result of my personal experience. In your moments of weakness, I hope you can draw on my story to provide you with hope, clarity, and a sense of optimism for a positive future.

References

Peris, Frederick. HOME. (n.d.).
http:littleblessings.me/

8

GATHERING THE CONFIDENCE TO ASK FOR HELP

> *"Sometimes good things fall apart so better things can fall together."*
>
> — *MARILYN MONROE*

I walked into the kitchen one night with my head held down after a day of heavy drug use only to meet my mom standing there. Taking a good and hard look at me, tears began to fill up in her eyes. The daughter she once knew was no longer present. She was medicated to the point of no return, feeling no pain. She grabbed my face as a concerned parent and pleaded with me to get myself help. Although it was just a seed she planted in my mind, I truly believed that help was not possible in that moment. I didn't think there could be reparation for the level of messed up that I had reached. I was on a suicide mission. I sedated myself as much as possible to get through the day. But I made sure my job was unable to notice because I remained as normal as possible. Looking back, I'm sure they knew by how red my eyes were and how my dark circles had receded to my cheek bone. They would drop hints that said they knew what I was up to. But the problem is I was so good at holding my feelings inside that everyone believed I was fine.

I felt like I was throwing my life away. That's because I was. I didn't know any other way than to self-sabotage. At the time, I was so ashamed to admit to my mistakes and stand in my truth.

Over the days, I began to take a harder look at myself in the mirror. The drugs were no longer helping me feel better. And I needed six to eight times the number of painkillers to feel like a normal human being. So when I would consume more than that, I just looked like someone I could no longer recognize. I had gone from an award-winning college student to an addict with severe mental health issues. Being diagnosed with Bipolar Disorder II when I was 19 years old, I did not understand the impact that my actions were having on destroying my life. At the time, I just believed I was better off numbing my emotions the only way I knew how. And for me, doing that helped me get through the day. Eventually, I became ashamed at the woman I had become. I kept this secret for so long, that it felt impossible to be honest about the real issues I was facing.

The more despondent and depressed I became, I started to plan how I was going to end my own life. I was going to take too many drugs and then drink myself until I never woke up again. I was planning on doing this one night after work. I had attempted suicide several times as a teenager but had never been successful. However, as the day went on, I decided to make some calls to clinics that might be able to help me immediately. I thought to myself, if someone could help, I might consider becoming sober. I made many calls.

By the last call, a nice and compassionate woman answered the phone. She made time for me the very next day. I was extremely grateful that anyone was willing to help.

By the grace of the angelic spirits looking out for me, I was able to get a ride from my boss at work. I pulled him aside to tell him I was struggling with serious depression and I needed help. He asked no questions and brought me to the mental health clinic. As he dropped me off, I was terrified to enter the building. In my mind, I was anticipating that no one was going to truly help me in the way that I needed. There is a big difference between getting an appointment and actually benefiting from mental health treatment - when I was a student at Rutgers, I had a good psychologist, but my psychiatrist did little to help me with a large majority of my issues. So, I smoked a quick cigarette and consumed the last bit of drugs that I had on me.

Once I stepped through those doors, I waited about 45 minutes before being seen. I paced back and forth still contemplating if I should walk out. And just as I was hitting the point of no return, the receptionist called my name. When I got to the back, I met a female mental health intake professional. She did a full mental assessment on me. When I began to share my story of all the traumatic events that were most affecting me, I choked on almost every word. It required immense effort to say the words that described the pain I had been enduring for so long. I talked about my mother's heart attack, my father's loss, my journey with sexual assault, and the near-death experience with my brother's girlfriend. The clinician was shocked to see that I had been holding on to this kind of pain and suffering without any coping skills to maintain them. She actually said that she understood why I did not want to live anymore. This, I believe, is rare for a counselor to admit. They rarely are honest about their personal opinions, but she was. Just feeling her level of compassion, honesty, and ability to listen made me feel like I had a chance for the first time in many years.

Just as I was about to leave, she dropped a bomb on me. She advised that I go to the mental health hospital for a few days so that I could stabilize my condition. Due to my inability to care for myself at the time, I agreed and signed the paperwork. I then immediately informed the boss that I would be staying. To my surprise, he was understanding and sympathetic to my situation. I was worried that I would lose my job. But knowing that getting help wouldn't cost me my job, helped me to feel secure about my hospital stay.

Soon, I called my mom and filled her in on the situation. It felt like hours until they arrived. My heart was thumping out of my chest and I had this sense of fearful optimism, as I waited for her to pull up. When she arrived, my stepdad was with her. I was grateful to see his support at this moment. But I couldn't tell him the real reasons why I was going to be admitted to the hospital. I wasn't sure how he would react to the fact that my hospital stay would be a mental one, not a physical one. To my relief, he said nothing. I was glad because I was not sure what explanation I had prepared for this moment.

The drive to the hospital was surreal. I felt like the scenery passing by was a warped figure of my imagination. My thoughts were in slow motion for the first time in months. I was speechless and not sure what to think. I genuinely believe mental exhaustion took over my body. For the first time in years, having my mom and my stepdad both in the same car during an urgent situation, I felt like my dad was back with me. I was grateful for the shared support and their willingness to do anything to ease my comfort in the moment. Although I assumed I would be going to the mental hospital first, I actually was going to the community medical center's mental health unit for further assessment. They re-evaluated me upon arrival.

Terrified by my own emotions, I realized it was now or never. Either I faced the truth and told it, or never get the help I needed. My shame could easily have held me back for the rest of my life if I'd let it. I distinctly remember three doctors gathering around my bedside, one man on my left and two women on my right. They poked and prodded, took blood samples, and did a full psychological evaluation. So when it came down to those glaring questions, I spilled the dirty truth. Upon asking me if I wanted to commit suicide, I told them I was going to that day, using a drug and alcohol overdose. Then when they inquired about if I used drugs, I told them yes. They began to dig deeper and I finally admitted that I had a problem.

I could have been dead by that point, but I chose to go to the mental health clinic as a last-ditch effort for help. I feel indebted to that woman who chose to listen to me when I was crying out and hyperventilating, struggling to get through my story. She believed I deserved the best treatment after all I had been through. To this very day, I believe she helped to save my life.

Since my case was so complicated, they sought to have a referral to a behavioral and mental health facility the next day. After giving them my all, I felt drained, but still agitated.

Once I was wheeled through the doors of this Barnabas Behavioral Health Unit, I was careful to remain quiet, to observe my surroundings in order to figure out my best course of action for my success. I'm pretty sure that's the student in me speaking. It was almost like I was trying to figure out the best strategy to ace this class. Only it wasn't a class, it was my real life in the hands of these strangers. I had to put my faith and trust in people I hardly knew, and it was hard for me to give up control over the situation. As I continued to look around, I realized that I looked terrible in comparison to the people walking back and forth for exercise enjoying what seemed to be an interesting conversation. I could tell that they had already been there for a few days because they looked more comfortable than me.

While sitting in the stretcher in the main entrance to the facility, I was told that I had to go for a full evaluation, which was the most degrading part of the whole experience. I was brought into this private room and told that I had to strip down naked. I was not thrilled at this since I had not been able to shower for the past day and a half. She went from head to toe and checked every single scar on my body and demanded an explanation for every single one. This is par for the course apparently, to make sure I had no current wounds hiding under my clothes. Then, the mental health portion began, where I was interviewed about why I was there. I told her that the recent traumas were too much to bear, in addition to my severe depression, mood swings, panic attacks, and flashbacks that occurred 24/7. I had lost control over my ability to deal. In fact, I didn't even understand what the word *coping skills* were. Growing up in a family that struggled with similar issues, I had not seen what was normal.

After being there about 7 hours, I began to settle in. However, I was still a little hesitant to deal with anyone yet. Not too long afterwards, they sent me to an in-house psychiatrist who started me on a series of medicines. Over the days, I kept trying different ones until I landed on the ones that helped me the most. The first night, rather than participating in any meetings they had going on, I went back to the room to sleep. I was not in the mood to face anyone just yet. I lay in the bed feeling so pessimistic about my recovery. I struggled to believe that these people could help me. That was another sign of my mental illness controlling the narrative. Little did I know, I had the power within me to change that. I just didn't have a reason to believe in myself yet. So I just followed what everyone else did for the first two days. By the third day, I started engaging in more social activities.

I remember the first meeting I went to. The group was discussing how to manage anxiety and stress in relation to drug use. And the resolutions seemed so simple. So why did I always struggle to calm down? As I observed the others in the facility, I learned a few things. First, I realized the power of my chemical imbalances were preventing me from achieving a sense of normalcy. Now that the medicines were leveling me out, I finally had the opportunity to work on acquiring coping skills, without these imbalances getting in the way. I also learned that I had to take responsibility for myself in order to remain successful in recovery.

During our six meetings a day, I became a sponge, working hard to observe as much as I could for the purpose of applying it to my recovery. As I sat there and listened, I realized that I was not alone. Everyone else there suffered from some sort of combination of mental health and addiction issues. I was nervous and sick to my stomach at all times because the withdrawals began to kick in. But some of the psychotropic medications kept me calmer than I would have been. Despite feeling as sick as I did, I made it my mission to speak at the first meeting. I didn't say anything too personal, but I thought trying to participate was better than being passive in my own recovery.

This was the first time I had taken responsibility for myself in public. I finally admitted I was an addict, struggling with many traumas. It seemed that after I spoke, others worked up the nerve to take the meeting seriously and share their stories. It was this one person's story that truly changed me. I am so grateful I had the chance to observe and listen in that moment because it was a major wakeup call for me. I realized why I wanted to die, and exactly why I should fight to live in the same moment. In addition, I considered that the turbulence and doubts in my head were self-inflicted. All these fears I have manifested were a direct result of my inability to see that I was capable of conquering and reconstructing the narrative in my mind.

So, this younger male was in his early 20s. He was the youngest man I had met who owned a large company that was going public. I was astounded to see such talent in someone so young. He seemed to have it all together, until he told his story. Between his words were signs of his compromised mental health slipping through the cracks. As he was becoming more successful, he stopped making time for self-care. This was single handedly his biggest mistake. As time went on, he stopped sleeping, eating, and working out. This is greatly detrimental to anyone's mental health, let alone someone with that level of pressure to remain responsible and successful on a regular basis.

Secondly, he placed no restrictions on work or private life. By allowing coworkers to contact him all hours of the night and day, he lost control of his own life. He basically gave the power within him to others so they could manipulate him like a puppet. Without making clear boundaries for what is okay and what isn't, people take advantage of our time. This comprises mental health greatly because then there is a lack control of what is acceptable, and what isn't.

For example, if you do not believe in answering the phone after midnight and value your personal time, frequent disruptions bring about immense stress. In instances where you are not comfortable being asked to get things done, even after making it clear you won't be able to do so, that is a prime demonstration of poor boundaries. Prior to this experience, I had no concept of what the term signified. But then I started to relate to this individual because I had recently been in a situation where I had given up all of my time to a job that left me with little free time to take care of myself. This greatly contributed to my mental breakdown.

It was that moment that I learned the value of starting over. I too wanted to die, just like this young man. He wasn't a drug addict, but he had similar issues. We both got so caught up in wanting to escape the torture of a tightly wound and controlled life, that we both lost perspective of what it meant to live. The verbs "to live" and "to exist" have different connotations entirely. All that time I had been existing as a puppet for others, instead of being clear that my time is my choice. And when I say it's time to take care of me, that should be respected. And those who do choose to disrespect me, do not need to be a part of my life, creating psychological distress for me.

The stories of several other members changed my

outlook on my own life. Hearing another person's struggles changed my mind about care-taking completely. There were many years I helped to care for my father, grandmother, and even my mother. I know how mentally taxing it can be. This is the danger of giving all of yourself to others without a border of self-care in between. During the middle of my stay, I heard this woman around the age of 60 years old bravely share to the group. She told us that she was an Alcoholic who struggled with the care of her adult daughter, who had mental disabilities.

To consider her point fully, I will say that most parents are done with the diaper changing and feeding after the first few years. I cannot imagine going through this for almost 30 years with a grown child. This woman's identity slowly disintegrated behind her husband's growing demands to put their daughter first and take care of him during his recent battle with cancer. Just imagining her anguish makes me bathe in sympathy and compassion. I can't imagine living my whole life, waiting to have that freedom to explore my older years, just to be tied down by immense burdens.

In order to deal with the daily adversities and lack of time dedicated to her own needs, she began to drink just to feel relaxed. This drinking created a boundary between her and her family, but not the good kind. Eventually, this drinking led to a complete disconnect between her expected role and her own desires. Her husband was so angry with her choice to even put her own recovery first, because of the daughter. This is a classic example of how boundaries can be violated by the selfish needs of others. If there is no self-care to protect and reinforce that line, there is no separation between one's needs and others. Even by the time I left, the mental guilt she faced still haunted her. I always wondered how she turned out. But now I can only hope that she has recovered a sense of peace and love for herself that can replace the guilt of being unable to put these unrealistic expectations first. I hope someone helps to remove the burden from her, by taking care of that child, so she has the chance to recover in an environment that is not the direct trigger for her drinking. I pray for her health, wealth, and recovery. I hope God is looking down on her, giving her the opportunity to smile at least once a day.

As the days reached their peak, I started to experience my worst withdrawal symptoms yet. I think it was because I had been clogging my body with all these substances for so long that it actually took a while to detoxify itself. When my symptoms became unbearable, my mental health struggled. I didn't believe that I could get through another moment without wanting to escape. I even had multiple mental breakdowns, almost requiring me to be sedated. But in those moments, the people that were in there with me rallied around me. Seeing them face their worst moments of withdrawal with me gave me a sense of courage that we could get through this together, even if we felt like it would kill us first. I would see that I had made it so many days when new people would be admitted, and I started to believe in myself more. The staff even stepped up to help me. They somehow saw the potential in me, and the academic I used to be was still there. I was *worth* salvaging, which is something I had not believed in a long time. I greatly appreciate all the individuals that came together on my behalf to make sure I made it through the worst days.

Throughout this experience, I realized that we all face our own hurdles in life. These are the reasons we choose to self-medicate, and drown out and numb our spirit with substances that prevent us from feeling. The world becomes so cold the instant we are forced to interact with its reality sober. Each day the layers of the Novocain cloak were peeling away from me, until I was finally forced to take an honest look at myself in the mirror. I would never be the same, so I would have to accept a new version of myself that made a bigger impact on this world. I had so many dreams left unrealized, so what was I waiting for?

It was that voice inside me telling me I was worth nothing for so long. I was waiting to be set free from that monster that left me chained to addiction. I just had to be willing to address all my self-created fears, then learn how to change them into positive action and reaction. If it were not for this experience, I would have never written this book or understood anything about my struggles with mental illness and addiction. Because of my choice that day, I have had the chance to start over. And for that, I am forever grateful.

So, when the last day arrived, I gathered all my belongings and met my mother at the front door. When I walked through the doorway and arrived on the other side, the fragmented parts of me began to heal as my new soul encountered the light for the first time.

References

A quote by Marilyn Monroe. (n.d.).
https://www.goodreads.com/quotes/12379-i-believe-that-everything-happens-for-a-reason-people-change

9

POST-REHABILITATION ADJUSTMENT

> *"Ya think that the Whiskey tastes good? Try a big cup of sobriety- now that's the good stuff!"*
>
> — *STEVEN TYLER*

The cloudy light that grazed my face was a sign that I was entering a new world of reality. I had clarity for the first time in a while. Without the toxic mind-altering substancces, I was able to see without those blurry goggles preventing me from seeing the beauty in the world. For the first time, I saw those clouds and did not have a negative reaction. Instead, I saw how I could turn this seemingly gloomy day into a positive for me. Although I was still feeling the lingering effects of the withdrawal, what replaced the physical weakness was a mental endurance that I used to have, way before I gave up on the concept of self-love and appreciation. I used to believe that the old me was gone forever. This was the first time in a while I had hope.

I thought to myself, I just have to peel back the layers of the dead onion that I have rotted away in the past few years. This is my way to start over. My next thought was, how do I succeed in an outpatient program? After my hospitalization, I was sent to Ocean Mental Health Center where I met with an intake counselor. I was required to provide my history of addiction, trauma, anxiety, depression, and mood instability. This woman, with the short hair and the big black glasses, saw through my bullshit excuses. So this lady told me, in order for me to receive ongoing care, I needed to sign up for the intensive outpatient care. I had heard from friends years ago that this is not an easy program to pass, because you are monitored for drug screens constantly and have to attend all sessions on time. I had no idea what I had got myself into. I was just terrified to have to go to this place where all the other disturbed individuals were. I was worried that working in a group long-term would prevent me from focusing on my own issues.

Boy, was I wrong. Upon attending the first day, I was told I needed to provide a monitored urine test. And yes, that sounds just as intimidating as it is. I struggled to urinate while someone was watching, waiting, and rushing me. After ten minutes, something finally came out! I was so relieved just to get it over with. So when my first urine came back negative for illicit substances and alcohol, I was proud of myself. This was now my second week of sobriety.

In those early days, I realized that those counselors did not allot trust to their clients - they had to earn it. The last thing I wanted to do was stay there forever. So, I stayed on the straight and narrow. I tried to be a "good" student. I participated, shared my deepest struggles to others in hopes that it would help me. But in return, I gained so much more. The more I gave to the group, the more they gave back to me in support, friendship, and guidance. I realized that we were all broken and had little trust. Because of that, we just couldn't do each other wrong.

I had started to engage in my individual counseling sessions. Although I didn't know it at the time, I had been set up with a compassionate counselor who would help me get to where I am today. She started to show that she believed in me. Even more so, she listened to my traumatic experiences and did not disregard me like other therapists had in the past. She helped me work on ways to deal with my emotions that did not include drinking or numbing the pain. I learned it was okay to feel, but there were better ways to process emotions. I had such post-traumatic stress disorder that I struggled for months to sleep properly. All the while, I learned how to live a substance free life.

So what does it really mean to live sober? For those truly doing it, it means something so much more profound. It's a lifestyle that is decided by choice, because we know internally, we cannot continue living the lives the way we used to. As addicts, we have to take control over our actions and daily decisions: to use, or to not use. For all those normal people out there, this is a simple choice. Yet for us, abstinence is the biggest struggle of all time. With our substance of choice, we have the ability to deal with all the pain, and bury it deep. We can function and live like nothing bothers us. When we do decide to abstain, we are left with all this TIME. So many hours of the day, that used to be accounted for, become eerily empty. These minutes are so packed with silence that we have all this time to drive ourselves nuts if we do not stick to something constructive.

Yes, living sober requires finding ways to replace empty time with self-work. However, that has to be done independently, and should be supplemented by a program of some sorts. This forces us to stay on track. We fill our days with group events and share feelings with other people who actually understand. And that's exactly what I did. I learned to enjoy reading again, taking care of myself, going to meetings, in addition to intensive outpatient care. I expanded my social networks and got a sponsor to help me on a regular basis. I knew that if I did not have daily guidance, it would be easy for me to just instantly turn my progress into failure and relapse. But for me, I refused to allow this to become a possibility. I promised myself I wasn't going to give up and have to go to rehab a second time. Besides, I promised my family. I knew my dad was looking down on me, waiting for me to make the right choices again.

I learned as much as I could from those mentors around me. Being honest with myself was the most important lesson I had learned. Without that, I could not gain the trust of the program counselors, sponsors, and group members. I knew I needed the help. I wanted to show them that I was worthy of receiving their time and wisdom.

Part of being honest with myself meant accepting my diagnosis. I was already familiar with the impact of my depression, anxiety, and mood instability. However, this new found interaction with post-traumatic stress disorder had left me stupefied. I had no clue how to stop the severe nightmares, the terrible memories, cold sweats, and dry heaving that were beginning to resurface. All that time, I had not come to terms with the fact that I even had an issue with PTSD. I always thought what I was going through was normal. I had lived with it for so long without knowing, so that's one of the reasons I drowned myself in addiction. Those substances helped me avoid the graphic and disturbing nature of my thoughts.

During my recovery, the medications I was prescribed helped me to remain calm enough to begin to address the entangled web of fear and trauma. The roots of my trauma ran so deep, that I didn't know where to begin. Because of this, I found myself each day struggling with a different part of my past.

HOW TO LIVE SOBER

When you think about it, it's a painful task to undertake. I was faced with attempting a level of discipline that even non-addicts don't have. One thing I have noticed over the years is that it doesn't require much encouragement to drink alcohol, even in the most unlikely environments. Or more often than not, people encourage this behavior as socially acceptable and normal. But to the individual that suffers with Alcoholism, making a mistake may be all too tempting.

Instead of giving myself too much slack, I decided it was best to have a self-talk, where I wrote a promise to myself. This almost served as an insurance policy for my failure. I made a deal with myself that said, "I promise to stay sober for at least the next year." Of course, during the first few months, I encountered difficulty because my emotions were no longer numb. The reality of all the pain I had been through hit me like a ton of bricks. Every day I was facing a new battle. In order to keep these raw painful memories at bay, I made sure to put all my time into therapy and the group work. The beauty of our differences is that they share one large commonality - our addiction. This was astounding to me - that everyone, from all ages and walks of life, could come together and listen to me with a sense of respect. And in return, I provided them with the same respect to ensure that we all worked in a non-judgmental environment. I wanted to make certain that our group was comfortable with each other. With each session, I started to see the real me, without all the substances, shine through. I had forgotten that person was still there at all. I hadn't wanted to be her anymore because that meant all that happened in my life was real. The part of sobriety that incorporated facing my true self was not grueling. I had to start introducing self-love after a series of anger and resentment for the past decisions I made.

So what does self-love even mean? I learned that it requires giving yourself acceptance and compassion in moments of emotional pain. Instead of being angry or judgmental, I learned how to speak to myself in a more gentle manner. I had to be a friend to myself, not my own worst enemy. When I needed time to take a break, I took it. I made a daily plan for managing my emotions as they surfaced rather than suppressing them.

Feelings are meant to become exposed, not hidden. The outcome of healing comes with properly acknowledging each emotional setback, rather than trying to prevent them from happening at all with drugs. By exposing these deep emotions to the light, they begin to degrade with time, just like how photos become lighter as a result of the sun.

This new awareness was monumental for me. If you are wondering what it means to live sober, this is it! It means learning how to feel again and being okay with you who are when you look in the mirror. You earn self-love and acceptance by releasing negative emotions deeply embedded under the surface. You even find the value in your weaknesses, become able to take responsibility for your flaws, and begin to work on them. The disclaimer that comes with this is: not every day will be easy, you have to find the positive aspect to every issue.

Some days you will feel like you got hit by a tractor trailer, and other days you will feel high off life. These valleys and peaks are natural, and are necessary for recovery. The moments of disruption and pain are signs of growth and change. Without these difficulties, it becomes clear you probably are not challenging yourself enough. During your low moments, it is necessary to lean on your therapist, sober coach, and fellow group members. They can prevent you from making mistakes by acting on your raw unprocessed emotions. By making your feelings known, they are spoken into existence. As a result, there is now the opportunity to work on tackling each disruptive fear emotion that may precede relapse.

Initially, I was afraid to get a sponsor. They are

mentors who help prevent their sponsees from engaging in substance use. Despite my hesitation, having one helped me remain accountable. Calling her daily and talking about my feelings prevented me from acting irrationally.

The first sponsor I ever had made the largest impact on me and is one of the main reasons why I am sober today. Because of her influence, I learned so much. Therefore, I feel it is my duty to share my knowledge with those who are still sick and suffering.

WAYS TO REMAIN SOBER

1. **Stay Busy:** If you do not keep yourself doing something productive, drugs and alcohol will inevitably invade your thoughts and try to convince you to go to the bar or call up your dealer. Remaining occupied is one of the most important things to do. My solution became going to *Alcoholics Anonymous* (AA) or *Narcotics Anonymous* (NA) meetings that follow twelve step programs for recovery. According to my experience attending these meetings, the ones that remain successful are those that remain connected with the other members with experience in recovery. It is easy to fall off if you isolate yourself. It is the biggest mistake you can

make in early recovery. If you need to find out where these meetings are being held, there are apps on the phone dedicated to finding the in-person or now, zoom meetings due to the Covid-19 pandemic. You can also spend time reading about topics that make you happy. The central idea is to not remain isolated in an unhealthy manner. For with a book, you are never truly alone. The books I have read during recovery have become my best friends. One of those books is the *Living Sober* book by Alcoholics Anonymous.

2. **Self-Care:** If you can't make a meeting, try to spend the time doing something positive for yourself, like getting a haircut, getting your nails done, reading a book, or exercising. This aspect highlights the benefits of self-care which must become a larger priority during recovery. One of the major problems about being an addict is that we have put so much time into trying to get our fix or release, that all other matters of our health and well-being fall by the wayside. For example, most people tend to neglect getting their teeth fixed, although these substances are causing them to rot out. So upon becoming sober, this starts to become a large priority because the pain is immense without all the painkilling

substances. Another problem that generally exists is not eating, this can lead to serious malnutrition and dehydration. The major take-away point from this section is to remember to take care of yourself in a way that boosts your confidence, eliminates stress, and makes you feel physically and emotionally at ease.

3. **Make a Journal:** I am sure this sounds like generic advice, but I promise it is actually worth your time. When I checked into rehab, I was forced to write in my journal daily. What is different about this journal from others, is that it will be focused on recovery. By doing this, I was able to identify the emotions that contributed to my drug use. I would even write creatively, which became a daily reflection of my anger, sadness, and depression. When I took a look at the weeks' worth of journaling, I was able to look at myself objectively for the first time, and see what everyone else was trying to say: I have been this doubtful girl, plagued by traumas. If I work on those issues, I have a better chance of recovery. The larger benefit is that I had a starting point to begin therapy, by keeping track of the biggest traumas that limited my ability to function as a normal human being.
4. **Lace Your Day with Positivity:** Being positive is

the most difficult thing to do as a person struggling with depression, anxiety, PTSD, etc. But this is critical to recovery as an addict. There has to be some acknowledgement of the fact that most of us project our day to be negative before it begins. In my life, one major source of negativity sounded like, "I know my day is going to be terrible. I'm not going to be able to survive it." This is what I would tell myself on the regular basis, not realizing that it is abnormal and counteractive to my progress. I learned about this in group therapy when the counselor asked how many of us have bad thoughts. One individual mentioned that their negative mindset stemmed from having more free time without chasing drugs all day. Because they were at home doing nothing, they felt useless. So the counselor responded by asking what this person could do to make their day more positive. The person said that they could spend that free time looking for a job. The counselor agreed that was a positive substitution for the expectation of a bad day being bored at home. She also said that changing our behavior could also be supplemented by a positive portrayal of the day ahead. She reframed his original statement with, "I believe I'll have a good day because I am being productive looking for jobs." In other words, it is not only the negative thoughts attached to your day, but also how you perceive the day before it begins. Both of these small changes lead to a major transformation in your thinking. It makes the world of a difference to project something good as opposed to believing the worst will happen.

5. **Making Short-Term Goals**: To coincide with believing in verbal presets for positivity, my group activities focused on formulating a giant list that displayed everyone's weekly goals. The primary intention is to build confidence and to reinforce positive thinking. When creating a small daily list, you can not only build up your self-confidence, but also put your life on track after being destroyed by addiction. The key to being successful with this is making sure that the goals can be easily accomplished, without the large possibility or expectation of failure attached to it. For example, you could take out the garbage and do the dishes. For those who would spend all day under the influence of drugs, their house was a mess. By introducing these small goals, there are vast alterations in habitual behavior. This ultimately serves as a reminder that you are capable of doing anything you put your mind to. The purpose of making

the list is to make sure certain more important goals are met over others that are not time-dependent. All of these daily and weekly achievements accumulate to a lot of measurable and demonstrable progress. Holding yourself accountable to do these small tasks over time helps you to trust yourself again when it comes to being a responsible adult.

6. **Daily Relapse Prevention Strategies:** In essence, this means making a daily routine of relapse prevention to ensure that you continue to grow and progress throughout early sobriety. There are an unlimited number of ways this can be organized and accomplished. As an addict in recovery, the number one thing that saves me from regressing, is having a daily procedure for my wellness. This is, of course, very individualized to your own unique needs. However, it is one of the reasons why I have remained on a good path where others I know have wavered in and out of rehab many times. Every morning, I make sure that my mental health comes first - for without that, I have no foundation for the day. I take my psychotropic medications to make sure I am stable at the chemical level. While the meds are kicking in, I take 15 minutes of quiet relaxation time with a

cup of coffee. For me, this serves as my form of meditation, where nothing else matters in that moment other than my mental peace. This prepares me for enduring stress at my job and the hostile, energy-draining people I deal with on the regular basis. Following that time, I would read my favorite book for 20 minutes to help me remain in a good mindset. Only after doing those self-grounding exercises, I would call my sponsor for the day. If any emotions were poking through that I just could not manage alone, I would bring them up. I would listen to her input and contribute my own solutions. The great part of speaking with someone about sobriety and mental wellness regularly is that you have the chance to bring your problems to light and offer healthy solutions to them. Thankfully, I was able to see the flaws in my own thinking and use that to my advantage by solving my issues without drugs, anger, or backlash on my loved ones.

SEEING THE SIGNS OF RELAPSE

Using the strategies mentioned above, these changes can become a new way of life. This becomes the foundation for creating coping skills that stick. Although it may take many tries to find out what works best for you, you have to try.

Without a daily habitual routine, it becomes a struggle to work through the AA, NA, or outpatient programs. As you grow in recovery, you can become aware of how to prevent backward movement in your journey. Part of the signs of relapse mean that those intrusive thoughts of negativity creep back in, along with the "I don't care what happens" attitude. This then becomes followed by prolonged and smaller deviations from the routine you have created for yourself.

Another major hurdle to overcome is dealing with major changes and crises during early recovery, like having to move, enduring a breakup, death of a family member, etc. Rather than allowing this to destroy everything you worked hard for, you must resist the urge to wallow in your sorrows. The best thing you can do is pick up the phone and ask for additional support. All of the numbers these counselors, NA, and AA members provide you with are intended to help you in those moments where you are on the verge of a mental breakdown and minutes away from relapse.

In those moments when you begin to question yourself and your ability to proceed down the path of positivity, I encourage you to do several things:

1. ***Make a Gratitude List*** -This entails making a list of all the things you are grateful for since becoming sober. For example, "I am grateful to

have my mom and brother by my side no matter what" or "I appreciate that I have a nice place to sleep and a roof over my head since many others do not."

2. ***Keep Fighting for Help!*** - One of the most important things to do is continue to fight for what you need in recovery. If you are crying out for help, ASK FOR IT. DO NOT STOP FIGHTING UNTIL YOU RECEIVE IT. This is the most crucial part of surviving this journey. If you do not vocalize your needs, no one will be able to rescue you from the pain. Besides, there are so many individuals who have been through similar situations. Just them being able to relate and offer their advice can be what you need to get back on your feet.
3. ***Do Not Self Destruct*** - It is so easy to criticize yourself and stop attending meetings and therapy. It won't be long before you feel the effects of giving up. Those people around you will try to help you resist doing so, so you have two choices: either stay off course or get back on track. If you make mistakes, it is okay, you are not perfect.

The next moment is another opportunity to do better. Do not allow your past imperfections define your present.

You have the ability to choose to do better at any time. Even after messing up by missing your day meetings, you can make the next one. If you missed therapy, reach out to your counselor, apologize and be honest. They will help you get back to the right frame of mind. So if you stop believing in yourself again, these professionals can witness the signs of your collapse before it happens. If you witness the early signs of self-destruction, you have the chance to intervene by requesting help before you relapse or stop taking your prescribed medications. It is necessary to listen to your feelings if they are amounting in a bad way because they can be lethal to your growth. Bad days happen, but do not let them accumulate without doing something about it.

References

Living sober. (1980). Alcoholics Anonymous World Services.

Ria Health (n.d.) 25 Recovery Quotes to Keep you Moving Forward. https://riahealth.com/2019/11/12/recovery-quotes/

10

PTSD & EPIGENETICS

> *"If the wounds on her heart and the bruises on her soul were translated on her skin, you wouldn't recognize her at all"*
>
> — *VERONA Q*

This chapter comes with a newfound sense of wisdom from great reflection. I have had so much time to think about all the contributing factors to my mental illness and PTSD. During the process of investigating my own life, and the information there about this trauma disorder, I have reason to believe that my inability to function normally may be related to my family history. From my generation to the previous three, many of my family members have struggled with a variety of issues, like chronic stress, depression, anxiety, PTSD, addiction, alcoholism. After speaking with my mother, the linkages between my environmental circumstances and genetics have played a large role in why I am who I am. This is not to say I regret or blame anyone in my family. Instead, I want to learn how I can break the cycle in my own life to prevent future generations from enduring the lethal combination of mental illness and addiction. As I have in my previous sections, I would like to explain these concepts in a manner that can be understood by everyone, with various forms of education, who come from all disciplines. To begin this segment, I will briefly explain what epigenetics is and how it interacts with PTSD. Then, I will describe how I believe these influences have affected my life.

WHAT IS EPIGENETICS?

Epigenetics is defined as the study of changes in organisms caused by modification of gene expression. As summarized by the Center for Disease Control (CDC, 2020), genetic changes can alter which protein is made, but epigenetic changes affect gene expression which controls what genes turn on and off. These modifications can happen by DNA methylation, histone modification, and non-coding RNA. The process of methylation refers to a group of proteins (methyl group) that attaches to the DNA to read the gene. The demethylation turns a specific gene on whereas methylation turns it off. Because DNA wraps around proteins called histones, DNA wrapped tightly around histones cannot be read by other surrounding proteins (Deans & Magger, 2015). The modification occurs in the way that some of the genetic sequences wrapped around histones cannot be interpreted and are turned off, while others are turned on. Lastly, non-coding DNA that is involved in altering sequences may recruit proteins to modify histones that either activate or deactivate certain genes (CDC, 2020).

I know this seems like technical terminology, but these terms are just complicated ways to describe how changes in and around genes occur. In order to get a better handle on this, I would like to better explain how epigenetics works.

If doctors need to determine someone's risk of a colorectal cancer, they might have to examine the changes in the genetic sequencing responsible for malignant cell metastasis. For this specific type of cancer, there is an increased methylation at the *SEPT9* gene. These changes can be uniquely identified using epigenetic-based tests that measure the methylation levels surrounding the *SEPT9* gene (Johnson et al., 2014; FDA, 2020). One way to measure changes in a given disease or illness may require examination of histone modification within certain subsets of cells.

WHAT IS PTSD?

As I have previously mentioned, I have struggled with post-traumatic stress disorder. At first, I failed to realize that I even had it. I had this abnormally large sense of fear and panic with simple interactions. For example, my earliest manifestation comes from one of my experiences being trapped in a closet. After my first interactions following the playdate gone wrong, I had flashbacks and cold sweats just going to other friend's houses. It was so bad that during every sleepover, I would have to call my mother to pick me up in the middle of the night. From there on out, I was convinced that almost every friend was going to harm me.

This panic, over the course of time, became much worse with the introduction of new traumatic experiences. It got to the point where I would dry heave, shake, and hyperventilate on and off for hours from a culmination of all my terrible memories. Each memory became so real in the moment that I thought I was truly being tortured over and over again. This became even worse in the recent years after the death of my father and the near loss of my mother. I had just no faith that the world was a safe place. In all my forms of panic, I was yelling but no one could hear me. It was as if I was screaming in the loudest silence possible. My disorder matured to the point where everything started to become a trigger for panic and avoidance, especially with situations that were new to me.

My goal here is to help those who are personally struggling with these issues as well as those who are trying to help someone else. But in order to truly understand the interaction between both PTSD and epigenetics, it is important to understand how panic manifests itself. From the behavioral level, this disorder is difficult to circumvent because of all the trauma associated with it and the myriad of symptoms that control a person's mindset. But for our purposes, it is helpful to refer to the clinical definition.

According to the American Psychiatric Association (APA), the definition of PTSD is:

A psychiatric disorder that may occur in people who have experienced or witnessed a traumatic event such as a natural disaster, a serious accident, a terrorist act, war/combat, or rape or who have been threatened with death, sexual violence or serious injury ("What is PTSD").

This association, using the Diagnostic Criteria version five as a reference, explains the four major symptom categories. The first one alludes to a concept known as *intrusion*, which refers to repeated thoughts or memories that become disturbing to the individual. These are also known as *flashbacks*. When these flashbacks occur, it feels as though the person is re-living the traumatic event over and over. A second common symptom with PTSD is *avoidance.* This consists of the affected individual intentionally trying to stay away from people, places, activities, or objects that serve as painful reminders of the traumatic event (Black & Grant, 2014). In accordance with these two major symptoms comes alterations in cognitions, mood, and physiological arousal. Distorted cognitions become linked to the event itself. Such as "because I was attacked by this man, all men should not be trusted" or "it's my fault that my father almost died." These thoughts become ongoing in a negative cycle that guide future actions and behavior. In addition, flashbacks associated with the original trauma may lead to permanent alterations in how someone behaves around other people. A person can remain in constant arousal, paranoia, and panic, leading to sustained elevation of heart rate and blood pressure. As a consequence, these individuals become overly sensitive to panic with future exposure to negative experiences.

Prior to learning more about this disorder, I was terrified by my own body. I believed that I was physically sick because I didn't understand why my body was reacting so robustly to normal stimuli. I just thought that I could sleep it off or control it with drugs. But the triggers were not only in my dreams. They surrounded me, threatening my ability to function like a normal human being in society. As a result of that, I became embarrassed to be around others. I started to isolate myself inside my room, and try to avoid contact with all people, and any situations that could be a trigger. Even worse, I knew that having too many friends would be a large problem because they wouldn't understand and judge me.

For me, I noticed the death of my father exacerbated my pre-existing issue with panic. I had nightmares of his death over and over. I could no longer sleep unless I drank a bottle of liquor. My stomach refused to tolerate any food and I could not talk to others because that meant bringing up his loss. And just the thought of relieving the moment of his death one more time was so excruciating that I thought I would lose consciousness. That's just one example of how robust these cycles of thoughts controlled my behavior and my physiological well-being. The avoidance became so strong that I could not go to, or even pass by the hospital where he died, and I struggled to look at pictures because I was too angry to accept that he left me. I didn't feel like I had enough time. We were just beginning to fix our relationship and I had just forgiven him for being an Alcoholic. It didn't seem fair to lose him when there was so much left for us to do together. Who would see me get married and walk me down the aisle? Who would be my first child's grandfather? No one. And the quiet behind those thoughts was devastating for me to fathom.

Just taking the time to seek therapy has led to this need to further educate myself. This started to set me free because I was starting to not be afraid of the flashbacks and the constant belly aching panic. I am convinced and certain that you can begin to overcome it if you also try to learn more about this disorder and how it came to affect you.

PTSD AND EPIGENETICS

The reason I am aiming to describe the linkages between PTSD and epigenetics is because I have noticed that poor coping skills, panic, depression, and PTSD come from my parents. There is experimental evidence to support this notion, which is why it has become a goal to explore in this section. A review article by Anthony S. Zannas, Nadine Provencal, and Elisabeth B. Binder (2015) explains the study of the epigenetics of PTSD. Epigenetic changes consist of various biochemical processes such as DNA methylation and hydroxymethylation, histone modifications, and non-coding RNA. These are all fancy terms to describe specific kinds of changes around genes. These specific processes have been shown to be influenced by exposure to different environmental stressors that change the transcriptional activity of the genes without altering the actual genetic code. Authors of this article mention that epigenetics brings the notion of nature versus nurture back into consideration, since the epigenome is an interface between the environment and the genome that can influence gene function and phenotypic expression. In other words, this concept demonstrates that the environment can affect expression of our genes, especially in circumstances of trauma. To support these claims, studies have found that combat veterans with PTSD have lower peripheral blood methylation levels compared to veterans who are not diagnosed with the disorder (Zannas et al, 2015).

Additional research reinforces the notion that PTSD can become learned within an individual and transferred throughout subsequent generations. Articles that study transmission of stress and trauma in Holocaust survivors demonstrate support for this concept (Kellerman, 2011; Yehuda et al., 2014). The article by Rachel Yehuda and Amy Lehrner (2018), describes how the children of these parents displayed severe psychiatric symptoms that would almost indicate that they were in direct exposure to those circumstances, even when the parents did not display any abnormal behavior. With regard to the Natan P.F. Kellerman article (2011), an evaluation of children of Holocaust survivors has reported they carry the emotional burdens of their parents through crying spells and the presence of fears that they were not originally exposed to. The possibility for transmission of fears and susceptibility to PTSD is passed down because the influence of environmental stress leaves certain marks on the coating or methylation of the chromosomes. In essence, this may become part of the latent memory within the cells (Van Der Kolk, 2015). This allows the children to become more vulnerable to remembering the stress of their parent's life during that devastating time period. Having the capacity for epigenetic cell memory may explain how specific elements of life experience are transmitted across multiple generations.

There is much more research that needs to occur before we are certain of how the process of epigenetics contributes to PTSD. Although this research is in its infancy, it has been life changing for me to learn about the linkages between my parent's exposure to trauma and how that increases my susceptibility. I believe understanding my role in this cycle is the key to creating a generation of better possibilities for my children and potential grand-children. If I am able to manage my battle with addiction, PTSD, bipolar disorder, and anxiety using the best methods available, future generations will have a better chance.

Because of my extensive history with trauma, this whole process of recovery has forced me to question how I got to this point. I mean, the intention is not to blame my parents or the other people in my life for their actions. None of my mental issues are their fault. I cannot blame them. What I can consider, is my family history with regard to my tumultuous development. Prior to starting this book, I often wondered what factors contributed to mental illness and how they might best be prevented. In order to do so, it is necessary to take a look at some of the traumatic events my family has endured. I will then compare it to my life and coping skills. Because of my understanding how epigenetics changes based on life experience, I have a lot of hope that if I turn my life around, subsequent generations will fare better in the long run.

CONTRIBUTING FAMILY HISTORY

For the purposes of my immediate comparisons, I will stick to the stories I was told by my parents. This allows me to have the information first hand in the most accurate manner in terms of emotional impact each traumatic event has caused. By speaking with my parents, I have quickly realized there are a lot of commonalities between my mother's life and my own.

First and foremost, my mother had a troubled past. She grew up in a bad neighborhood in Newark, New Jersey, where there was lots of violence. With even the most loving mother and a family of six children, there was only enough money and resources to go around. Unfortunately, mom grew up only meeting her father several times. For her that was pretty much like not having one at all. Her living situation was complicated by a need to protect herself at all costs, fighting off gang violence, taking a bullet, and having to live like an adult from a young age. Besides those daily stressors, she had endured several major losses in her life. Her brother committed suicide and so did one of her good friends. This changed the way she perceived the world. Pain became a replacement for hope and optimism. She learned firsthand how daily stressful experiences altered her ability to cope properly. The constant stress, danger, and violence in my mom's adult life has permanently altered the way her brain operates. Since her environment was dictated by these bad experiences, she learned to expect them and those changes became etched into her biochemical processes.

My father on the other hand, was a Vietnam War veteran who battled with PTSD for most of his life. Prior to joining the marines, he had already been a victim of gang violence, traumatic loss, and family addiction. Upon going to war, his problems became magnified into a major drug habit that was hard to break. His pain was managed by drugs and alcohol because he too inherited these vulnerabilities to anxiety, depression, panic disorder, and PTSD. This is a direct result of his own father being a war veteran, as well and his mother enduring a massive brain tumor that took her life. The previous generations did not live without these massive traumatic events. And it is my belief that I have become sensitive to these mental health disorders and addiction because of the previous generations. In other words, their brains endured genetic changes that were then passed on to me. As a result, it did not take much exposure to painful experiences before I too was suffering with mental health conditions, amplified by addiction.

BREAKING THE CYCLE

After learning about how PTSD and trauma can become an intergenerational problem, this has forced me to consider how to prevent my future children from enduring the same issues. In order to do so, I must take action in my own life so that these biological markers are no longer leaving a scar on my genes. By working hard to overcome my panic disorder, anxiety, and depression, my children will have a better chance to succeed. They will also be able to have a mother with the proper set of coping skills and positive mindset that they can use to flourish.

The next and final chapter will address the major concerns raised so far. First, I will discuss how to recognize your fears and overcome them, incorporating a process used from my own therapy sessions, plus my own personal experience with the matter. Then, I will discuss how to use fears as a springboard to living a life unhindered by these hesitations.

References

Black, D. W., & Grant, J. E. (2014). *DSM-5 guidebook: The essential companion to the Diagnostic and statistical manual of mental disorders, fifth edition*. American Psychiatric Publishing.

Deans, C., & Maggert, K. A. (2015). What Do You Mean,

"Epigenetic"? *Genetics, 199*(4), 887-896. doi:10.1534/genetics.114.173492

Johnson, D. A., Barclay, R. L., Mergener, K., Weiss, G., König, T., Beck, J., & Potter, N. T. (2014). Plasma Septin9 versus Fecal Immunochemical Testing for Colorectal Cancer Screening: A Prospective Multicenter Study. *PLoS ONE, 9*(6). doi:10.1371/journal.pone.0098238

Post-traumatic Stress Disorder. (n.d.). https://www.apa.org/topics/ptsd

Kolk, B. V. (2015). *The Body Keeps the Score*. Penguin.

What Is Posttraumatic Stress Disorder? (n.d.). https://www.psychiatry.org/patients-families/ptsd/what-is-ptsd#:~:text=Posttraumatic stress disorder (PTSD) is, sexual violence or serious injury.

What is Epigenetics? (2020, August 03). Retrieved from https://www.cdc.gov/genomics/disease/epigenetics.htm

Yehuda, R., & Lehrner, A. (2018). Intergenerational transmission of trauma effects: Putative role of epigenetic mechanisms. *World Psychiatry, 17*(3), 243-257. doi:10.1002/wps.20568

Zannas, A. S., Provençal, N., & Binder, E. B. (2015). Epigenetics of Posttraumatic Stress Disorder: Current

Evidence, Challenges, and Future Directions. *Biological Psychiatry, 78*(5), 327-335. doi:10.1016/j.biopsych.2015.04.003

Declutter The Mind. (2021, February 27). 100 PTSD Quotes to Help You Cope With Trauma. https://declutterthemind.com/blog/ptsd-quotes/

11

LIVING FEARLESSLY

"Becoming fearless isn't the point. That's impossible. It's learning how to control your fear, and how to be free from it."

— *VERONICA ROTH, DIVERGENT*

After writing about and reviewing the origins of my most painful fears, such as love, loss, abandonment, and success, I have learned that going back to the beginning is merely the first step. After doing so, you must consider what damage or mark these traumatic events have left on your life. For example, my first experiences with distrust in friendship has led me to believe that people cannot be trusted. Then the loss of my first home and my most loved family members has resulted in me expecting to lose everything that I cared for deeply. In reality, these are constructs that my mind has created to rationalize and explain why all these bad things were happening. But the truth is, I was the one making myself believe, for all these years, that I would not be happy because I would lose everything I loved and I would not be successful because I wasn't good enough. These are the flaws in my thinking that I am taking the time to highlight. Being a trauma therapy graduate, I have been able to look back at these experiences and understand that I am in the driver's seat when it comes to my own happiness. I have the power to become less depressed.

In order to take back the control of my life, I had to take responsibility for what I was doing wrong. As my therapist has described to me, when it comes to PTSD and fear, there is a strong sense of avoidance that predetermines our actions, thoughts, and behavior. In other words, we will work hard to make sure that whatever it is that hurts us stays far away from our daily lives. For most of us, this is not a healthy way to live. We cannot just avoid everything because we have been hurt before. Yet most of us have certain issues that cause us to hide. This can manifest in many forms. Namely, my largest problem with love was allowing my heart to be open rather than using men to fulfill my physical needs. Because of being assaulted, I was afraid to be kissed on the mouth because I kept seeing my attacker's face and tasting his breath. This has been hard to overcome until I not only talked about it, but told my story over and over in therapy. It caused me to think about and face the pain until it no longer hurt me. This is referred to as *prolonged exposure therapy.* Each time I would tell my story, I would rate my level of disturbance. The goal was to desensitize myself to the event over the course of time until I was able to think, talk about it, and continue my personal relationship with my boyfriend in a healthier fashion.

For me, exposure therapy has been entirely successful in allowing me to live a normal life again, where I can be my unhindered self. Despite this therapy, there was other work that I had to do to make improvements in my life as a whole. Furthermore, there are other effective methods for addressing these specific problems. Ultimately, I hope that you can learn from my experience. My hope for you is to live a life where your past no longer dictates your present. In order to do so, I will provide a concise list of steps towards living fearlessly.

HOW TO CONQUER YOUR FEARS

1. **Reviewing the origin of the fear:** As I have previously mentioned, the first step is to figure out which events have started affecting your life. This section is called finding and assessing the

damage that these traumatic events have had on your life. For this step, all you need is a pen and paper. Write down your fears on the left side and the first time they emerged on the right side. If you choose not to do this, it will be difficult to see why your life has become this complicated mess. This is the most important stage.

2. **Perform background research:** Learning about the object of our fright leads to less anxiety. This advice falls in line with the previous sections of my book where I took the time to research the issues I was struggling with. For example, I battled symptoms of chronic grief and the quality of my life was deteriorating. So, I took the time to read information online about why this happens from not only the clinical, but also from the scientific perspective. Doing this helped me to see the bigger picture. I realized that I am not alone, and many other individuals are enduring the same battle with the loss of a loved one. This is actually so much of a concern for psychiatrists that it is even mentioned in their diagnostic manual. I was finally able to see that I was not going insane. Instead, what I was going through was more common than I thought and there were medical and therapeutic options out there for me if I could not get better on my own.

Taking the time to learn about these issues can help you to know whether or not it is appropriate to seek professional help or consider psychotropic medications. In my case, I did need outside care and I never would have reached out if I didn't take the time to understand that my symptoms were just beyond basic self-care.

3. **Traumatic Events Are the Exception, NOT the Rule:** For those of you who suffer with mental diagnosis such as anxiety, depression, bipolar, or PTSD, there is one misleading conception that prevents you from making progress. That is, the outstanding belief that one or several tragic events will be the outcome for all future occurrences. In other words, if you were attacked one night on the street while walking home alone, this does not mean that you will probably be attacked every other time you're by yourself in the dark. This is how we tend to justify the worries that take control of our thoughts and behaviors. Rather than feeling safe, we feel constant panic brought on by this first event. Then this becomes complicated by avoiding walking alone at all at night. As this panic progresses, it will generalize to other circumstances such as being alone during the day, not just walking but in your car or in the

store. These thoughts can be intrusive and counterproductive. Before you know it, you will not be the fun-loving person you once were.

4. **Address the Cognitions That Define the Fear:** One you realize that you possess the potential to face your fears, your negative irrational thoughts must be targeted. Take that same piece of paper that contains your list of fears and make a separate page for all the thoughts and beliefs that surround each one. When I performed this activity, I realized that there were many terrible thoughts limiting my happiness. I wrote down thoughts such as, "I will never be loved because everyone is always trying to hurt or take advantage of me!" Another one was, "I am never going to be good enough no matter how hard I work."First of all, this is not a rational statement. In the real world, this is a statement filled with falsehoods. More likely than not, I will interact with others in a way that does not hurt me. The only thing that makes me believe this nonsense is myself. What already happened partially did so because I did not create safe boundaries and gave too much of myself to those around me. This ultimately led to others taking advantage of me. As a consequence, my sense of self-worth dwindled. The more that I recognized just how

obtuse my thinking was, the more I could change. This is what I want you to recognize within your own lives. There are many instances where your cognitions are having a counterproductive influence on your life.

5. **Identify Your Problematic Behaviors:** Now that you are finally identifying your problematic thoughts, it is time to work on what you have physically done to reinforce your negative thinking. This is a one day at a time approach. Once you have taken note of your flawed thought processes, you will need to identify the behavior that is linked to them. Continue with your previous notes by recording your actions that correspond to your thoughts. For example, along with the statement "I will never be good enough no matter how hard I work," I realized that I do not always put my full effort because I believe I am inferior to others, from my past experiences. I also have learned that I am afraid to be too confident since my experience with my senior thesis in college where everyone around me expressed immense doubt and discouragement. These elements of behavior are important to consider, especially when you take the time to work on changing them. Do not hold back when completing this step. It is critical to

be as honest with yourself as possible. This is the only way that you can make genuine improvements.

6. **Forgive Yourself for Your Shortcomings:** Forgiveness is a crucial part of healing from battle wounds. Without taking the time to tackle my anger, frustration, and lack of belief in myself, I would not be writing this book. I was in a dark place mentally because I believed my life would be significantly better if I had done certain things differently. But the truth is, I am living in the present moment. I cannot go back to what once was. Because I lack the control, I must learn to accept my imperfect thoughts, behaviors, and decisions in those moments where my paralyzing fears emerged. The best way to accomplish self-forgiveness is to apply self-love in those moments there is pain, anger, or regret. When I look back at my worst life events, I was in a different mindset and perspective. So, I must learn to love that previous version of me that was more naive. I cannot fault my 16-year-old self for not screaming loud enough during my assault. I was terrified to use my own voice to protect myself. It has taken lots of therapy and independent work, but I can finally look back at that time without regret. I

did the best I could to protect myself. I know that for certain and there is no more anger and regret surrounding myself on that day. If you want to forgive, you also need to replace anger, regret, and pain with self-love and compassion.

7. **Forgive Those Who Hurt You:** The second part of this process requires taking the perspective of those that hurt you. When I was attacked, I did not understand why. I went through intense shame from being taken advantage of and saw this man as the enemy. Not until recently have I learned that I should try to see the world through his eyes. Understanding him and his background helps take the blame off of myself and my attacker. When I think back to the situation, I knew that he struggled with drug addiction, grew up in a bad neighborhood, and had bad friends to influence him. He might have also struggled with self-esteem issues because of his awkward appearance. Therefore, the attack may not have been about me at all. It was more about being in control of his own life for a moment. Because of his upbringing and bad influences, I believe he was destined to be a criminal in some fashion. Being able to understand the contributing factors has allowed me to forgive him for attacking me because I

> understand why he did it. I cannot be angry anymore. He had done this to other girls as well, so I know that I was not the only target. He had his own mental issues that caused him to do what he did to me. There was nothing I could have done to change that. As a result of making these considerations, I have been able to forgive not only myself, but my attacker as well.

FORGIVENESS TAKES TIME

Once you take the time to notice the errors in your cognitions and behavior, you can learn how to take time to forgive yourself and others. This allows you to move forward with the healing process. However, I do not expect this part of the process to be easily accomplished. Even if you cannot reach forgiveness, you can come back to this step after working on how to change your thoughts and behaviors rather than just recognizing that they are troublesome.

After working these steps, I will show you how to incorporate the elements of this book into a new 7-day plan to positivity. This strategy is aimed to get you actively working on having a better mindset to combat your painful past. By improving your mindset, you are on your way to living a peaceful existence, where what happened can no longer harm you. This is the next phase, after identifying all the preliminary work I describe. I hope you can use this plan as a starting point for your progress.

THE 7-DAY PLAN TO POSITIVITY

As I have briefly mentioned in earlier chapters, there is a specific process that I have used to prevent the negative thoughts from dominating my mind. This method has also worked for those that made this journey of recovery with me in the mental health facility I attended two years ago. Reflecting on my experience, I will explain my 7-day plan to take charge of your life and the recurrent patterns of pessimistic cognitions that prevent your productivity. I will also describe what strategies to employ to make these immense improvements. It may seem that your hope is dwindling, but this is not true. Where there is pain, there is opportunity for change.

Days 1 & 2

Because these are your first days making the attempt to change, you must remember to not be hard on yourself. On these days, you are taking inventory of the powerful thoughts that decrease your levels of optimism. What's different about this from the previous exercise is that this involves reinforcing the work you have done identifying the thoughts and behaviors surrounding your fears. Only this time, the same method will also be applied to the rest of your issues such as self-confidence, depression, body image, etc. This casts a wider net to include all flawed thinking because the changes you make have to be applied throughout all aspects of your life.

To begin the first day, open your notebook where you wrote down how you talk to yourself about your fears. On the back of the same page, describe all other intrusive thoughts that consume your mind on the regular basis. This process is not immediate, it takes a couple days to consider and take responsibility for what damaging words you say to yourself. So, feel free to take your time with this first segment. If you cannot acknowledge the errors in your cognitions, it is nearly impossible to continue the rest of the process.

Day 3

Neutralize The Negativity

This is the day that you will begin to work on transforming those poisonous thoughts into ones less damaging to the psyche. As mentioned in a previous chapter, I challenge you to change or neutralize every statement you wrote with a negative connotation. This can be quite demanding for those of you enduring a long battle with mental health diagnoses. Starting out with your fears, you must reframe the personal statements to reflect neither a positive or negative meaning.

Ex 1. "Everyone hates me because I am ugly and fat," you can say, "Being larger in size makes me different, but not hated by those around me."

Ex 2. "Every time I walk alone, I believe I will be mugged" can be changed to, "Walking alone does not necessarily mean I will be attacked."

The trick to making improvements here is to target the key words that are signals of cognitive distortions, such as 'never, everyone, every time, and always.' These words are used to describe extremes, which largely distorts reality. Furthermore, thoughts can be neutralized by making unfounded assumptions about what you believe will happen based on your bad experiences in the past. Another distortion may appear in the form of large generalizations that occur on the basis of a one-time event. Just because one man was abusive to you, this does not mean all men will be the same way. It is unbeneficial to use these distortions because they lead to maladaptive patterns of thinking.

Day 4

Transition From Neutral to Positive

This day involves a similar method as the previous day, only the degree of change you're aiming for is greater this time, because for those of us that struggle with varying degrees of mental illness, it is often hard to make the transition from negative to neutral territory. Once you have accomplished those goals on day three, I am here to encourage you to take your progress another step further. Today you have to change your neutral thoughts to those that are filled with positivity. The aim is to remain realistic; NOT just make something up to make yourself feel better.

Ex. 1 "I will never be loved," to "I am worthy of being loved because I am beautiful inside and out". What makes this phrase positive is by removing the extreme language such as the word 'never.' These end all be all words are exchanged with the positive form of the sentence followed by an *explanation* that includes a *positive affirmation*. This is a fancy term that describes a statement which declares a truth or reinforces why something is true.

Ex. 2 "I am a loser and always will be" can be changed to, "I am a winner because I have survived the worst with all odds against me!" During this process, I highly encourage you to write the opposing form of the sentence reinforced by a truthful explanation. By working on changing all the statements from your original list, you become a firsthand witness to your own self-destruction. Having this major epiphany allows you to realize that you have the ability to become happy, if you take the time to replace all your negative and false thoughts with those that are true.

After completing these exercises, it is necessary to continue practicing on your own without using the worksheet. You must continue to catch yourself engaging in this discouraging self-talk and then practice the alternative solution (making the transition to positivity).

Day 5

Engage In Tasks That Reinforce Positive Thinking

As you begin to realize the power lies within you to change, you will consider how to become unhindered.

Day 6

Reward Yourself with Praise

Once you have begun to make progress in your 7-day plan, you must find ways to reward your hard work. Otherwise, it may feel like you put in all this effort for nothing. One of the best things you can do for yourself is improving your self-care. You can take the time to draw a bubble bath, do a face mask, paint your nails, do a deep conditioning treatment for your hair, and even take a couple days off from work. Another way to do this would be to praise yourself with material items. You can buy yourself that shirt you've always wanted after several successive days of positivity. Make these short-term goals that you can accomplish so that you can continue to have reasons to reward yourself.

The note of caution that I have is this: it is okay to have bad days in this process. There will be moments where everything you practiced goes out the window. If that happens, take the time to regroup and pick back up the next day where you left off. Besides, each day is a fresh start and, in this process, you have to leave the bad days where they belong otherwise, they will continue to haunt you and stunt your progress.

Day 7

Your New Life Begins

If you have made it this far, I am handing you a huge congratulations! This is a major accomplishment. You will notice as time goes on that your old behaviors will begin to vanish as your new mindset becomes habitual. The giant leash of negative thoughts held you back from being your true self and now that you have severed the restraints, you can live an unfettered existence. You will no longer be bound by the chains of your traumatic past and you will find yourself getting a better handle on any pre-existing mental health issues.

I am proud of you for taking these steps seriously and taking back control over your own life, rather than allowing your fears, doubts, and pain to tell you how to live. Thank you for making time in your life to read my story and particiFe in my steps to success. I promise that you will be feeling much after putting the work in. Overall, I am grateful for my bad experiences because I learned so much from them. In reality, if I endured nothing painful, I would not be here writing this book to help others. No matter how hard it has been to be entirely honest, I am glad I bared it all so that those who are struggling with the same issues have the chance to succeed, and even surpass me.

I want to say thank you to my therapists for believing in me and not allowing me to give up on myself. And I am especially in debt to my family and boyfriend who have supported me throughout this entire process. Like a monologue in acting, there were so many fears I told myself I could not overcome. But at the end of the day, I am the living proof that you can be afraid of so many things and still end up living a fearless life. So I know that you can do it too, if you believe in yourself and put in the hard work. Keep your head up and take it one day at a time and you too will be living the life you always dreamed of.

I know these steps may seem impossible to accomplish, but I want you to know that I believe you can do it. Your life of fear has a resolution. You just have to be willing to do the work. Then one day, you will be graced with a level of peace you've never experienced.

References

Fearless Quotes (728 quotes). (n.d.).
https://www.goodreads.com/quotes/tag/fearless

ABOUT THE AUTHOR

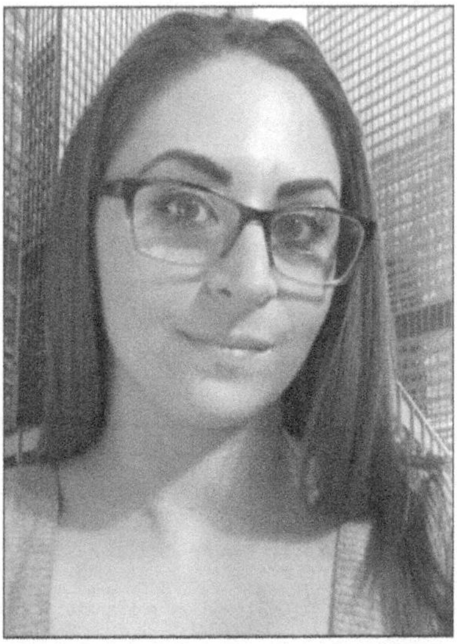

As a three time scholarship award winner, founder of Carla's Psychology Blog, and owner of a content writing agency, Carla M. Ralston has helped many students and professionals to harness the power of their voice through writing.

Graduating from Rutgers University with a Bachelor's degree in Psychology, Carla has used her academic experience to jumpstart her blog and business to educate about mental health, trauma, and addiction.

If you would like to become a ***featured writer*** for her website, learn how to cope with a mental diagnosis, or participate in her educational community,

please visit: carlaspsychblog.com or contact: carlaspsychblog@gmail.com

Follow us on Instagram at

instagram.com/carlaspsychblog

Made in United States
Cleveland, OH
05 November 2026

47667142R00143